THE
CHOOSE
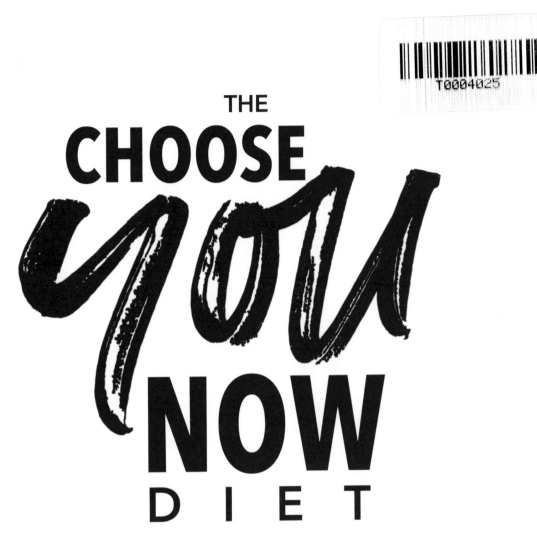
you
NOW
DIET

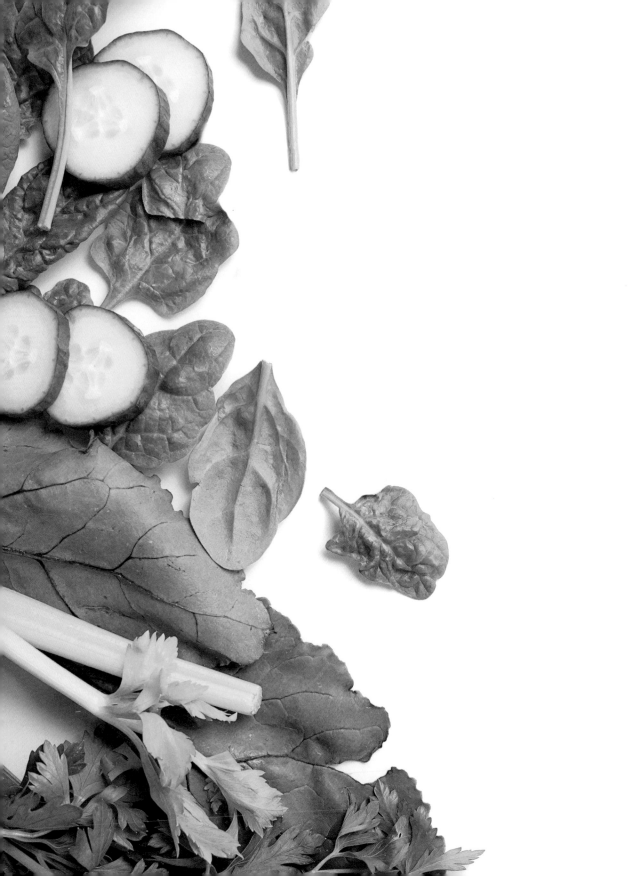

THE
CHOOSE
You
NOW
DIET

Julieanna Hever

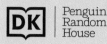

Publisher Mike Sanders
Editor Ann Barton
Designer and Art Director Rebecca Batchelor
Photographer Kelley Schuyler
Food Stylist Lovoni Walker
Chef Ashley Brooks
Recipe Tester Patricia Malone
Proofreaders Lisa Starnes, Monica Stone
Indexer Celia McCoy

First American Edition, 2021
Published in the United States by DK Publishing
6081 E. 82nd Street, Indianapolis, IN 46250

Library of Congress Catalog Number: 2021942879
ISBN: 978-0-7440-4435-5

Note: This publication contains the opinions and ideas of its author. It is intended to provide
helpful and informative material on the subject matter covered. It is sold with the
understanding that the author and publisher are not engaged in rendering professional
services in the book. If the reader requires personal assistance or advice, a competent
professional should be consulted. The author and publisher specifically disclaim any
responsibility for any liability, loss, or risk, personal or otherwise, which is incurred as a
consequence, directly or indirectly, of the use and application of any of the contents of this
book.

Trademarks: All terms mentioned in this book that are known to be or are suspected of being
trademarks or service marks have been appropriately capitalized. Alpha Books, DK, and
Penguin Random House LLC cannot attest to the accuracy of this information. Use of a term in
this book should not be regarded as affecting the validity of any trademark or service mark.

DK books are available at special discounts when purchased
in bulk for sales promotions, premiums, fund-raising,
or educational use. For details, contact:
SpecialSales@dk.com

Printed and bound in China

All images © Dorling Kindersley Limited

For the curious
www.dk.com

The Choose You Now Diet is dedicated to our magnificent bodies. Our bodies that keep our hearts beating; our lungs filling with air; our hormones flowing as needed; and our circadian clocks intimately tied to daily, monthly, and seasonal patterns without any conscious work on our parts. Our bodies that walk us through life and enable us to smell roses; feel rain; bond with an animal; watch a sunset; and experience love, pain, joy, heartbreak, excitement, disappointment, successes, failures, wins, losses, and passions. These same extraordinary homes we live in from birth to death, that know how to fight off microbes and inflammation and stress; that tap into our fat storage when we run low in glycogen, and that hold onto fat in order to survive in times of scarcity. You just need to let your naturally brilliant body do what it is programmed to do. Step out of its way, and experience gratitude and love for your inner wisdom. Nourish your body and your mind. You already know what you need to do.

Contents

Plates 102

Power Bowls 126

Secret Sauces 150

Foreword

If you have opened this book with any or all of the following questions in your mind,

"How do I begin to eat more healthfully?"

"How do I lose weight without being hungry all the time?"

"What if I fail or fall off the wagon?"

"What will my friends and family say?"

"How can I be sure I'll succeed?"

then you are holding the answers right in your hand.

In these pages, Julieanna Hever, registered dietitian, plant-based author, and health coach *extraordinaire,* shares her experienced guidance with all the qualities of a great coach.

Like any great mentor, she places the responsibility for healthy eating and practical food preparation squarely in our hands. Who else is going to help us get healthy, but us? After all, the diet is rightly called the "Choose You Now Diet," and she makes it clear that the first step toward creating a healthy body—and a healthy future—is to actively *choose ourselves* as the ones who will create and receive the gift of healthy, plant-based eating.

Then, rather than just presenting cold, hard nutritional facts, Ms. Hever equips us for success using the qualities of a truly great coach:

- compassion, as she has been a beginner herself
- empowerment, as she shares the keys to help us grasp the main principles of healthy eating
- wisdom, as she equips us with tools to help reap the lessons from mistakes while not being injured in the process
- patience, as she knows that making mistakes and trying again are essential to learning
- determination, as she knows life is lived one day at a time and that mastery is acquired through one conscious action after another, repeated lovingly over time

All these qualities imbue Ms. Hever's writing on every inspiring page.

The Choose You Now Diet is chock-full of practical information to make shopping, cooking, and even eating out in restaurants logical and health supporting. From batch-cooking suggestions that minimize food preparation to the smart use of frozen foods and staple ingredients to get food on the table quickly and deliciously, this book offers the keys to creating a maximally healthy body with a minimal amount of time and hassle.

Julieanna even devotes space to psychological techniques to fortify you against moments of temptation and backsliding. *The Choose You Now Diet* is a book for our times written by a teacher and dietitian for our times. Choose to read this book now, and you will choose healthy and delicious eating for a lifetime. I assure you, you will be in good hands for the journey.

Michael Klaper, MD
Director, *Moving Medicine Forward Initiative*
Author, *Vegan Nutrition: Pure and Simple*

Introduction

My Journey

Many lifelong personal circumstances led me to pursue the "secrets" of weight loss. I was raised in Los Angeles–the epicenter of emphasis on physical appearance–and body image has always brought with it an unignorable pang. This is a loaded idea, as it is undeniably a luxury to even have this as a concern. It is a blessing to live in an environment with adequate food to eat, to generally be healthy, and to live in a safe-enough nook of the world that body image can even matter. And yet, within that microcosm, with the naivete of a young girl, it fueled my desire to understand and solve this problem.

I began dancing before I could walk, according to my mom, and spent many years in ballet and other dance. When I was around 10 years old, my body started changing–changes that were witnessed during the hours spent in front of the mirrors in dance class practicing *pliés, tendus,* and *pas de bourrées.* One day, my teacher called out in front of the class, "It's time to cut out your snacks, Julieanna." I wanted the floor to swallow me and make me disappear. I began my obsession with diet and hating my body right then and there. I spent the next years experimenting and exploring, full of self-recrimination and frustration.

During my teenage years, like many in Los Angeles, I was an aspiring actress. I attended a performing arts high school (much like the television series *Fame* in the 80s), performed and toured with a couple theatre companies, and auditioned and worked a bit in television and film. I had agents and managers, headshots and auditions; and endured the bombardment of people telling me I was too fat or too thin, too brunette or not brunette enough, too tall or too short, too talented or not talented enough. When I showed up to auditions–especially for commercials or modeling–the other candidates all looked eerily similar. We were all brunette, around 5 feet 4 inches tall, and have similar features. But the worst of these experiences for me were when my manager or agent reminded me I needed to lose weight, "Just a few pounds. For the camera." It was as though my career and my acceptability in the world were based on a number on the scale and how I looked.

Ironically, this discovery did not lead me on an unrelated career path. I did not become a lawyer or accountant, as my dad so deeply wished for me. Instead, I decided to become a personal trainer, so I could learn all the secrets to achieving and maintaining a healthy, fit, and strong body without a constant struggle. Despite leaving acting in search of pursuing a path to help others who had struggled with their weight, once again, people decided whether to take me seriously after looking me up and down to determine how I managed my body shape and size. And I didn't stop there. When I began training clients and they persistently asked me what they should eat, I was certain I did not want to simply recite facts I had memorized in my personal trainer handbook or from the hundreds of books I had studied over the years. This was my opportunity to really dive into the science and finally find the secrets that I knew must be hidden somewhere. I applied to graduate school to become a registered dietitian and pursue a master's degree in nutrition. Surely, I would get to the bottom of the conundrum of easy, healthful, sustainable weight management and then be enabled to help others resolve their struggles once and for all.

Well, decades later, after studying and seeking, digging and discovering, prodding and practicing; I can honestly say there are no secrets. We are human after all.

Our Humanity

Losing weight is not fun. Inherently, the process is not entertaining, sexy, or pleasurable. No matter how you approach it, a deficit must be created in order to tap into the body's energy storage organ—*adipose tissue*, also known as "body fat." Our bodies brilliantly evolved to store energy when confronted with calories because calories were not always available, and there were often stretches of time when food was scarce. This is a powerful—and essential—survival mechanism. Now, that evolutionary advantage exists in a society where abundance dominates—where there is not only access to food at all hours of the day, but there are messages of enticement that are unavoidable. We are bombarded with gratuitous commercials for cheesy, decadent pizzas; sugary, fun breakfast cereals; and dollar menus offering extraordinary amounts of cheap calories packaged with hyperpalatable dopamine hits and their associated health-damaging sequelae. Even worse is the final piece of this abundance triad: the normalization of food overconsumption. Not only is it normal to eat and normal to indulge in less than optimal food, but it is abnormal if you decline the opportunity. Saying "no thank you" to dessert, or "I'm not hungry," or "I'm on a plant-based diet" is considered extreme and socially inappropriate or awkward. We eat to celebrate, to mourn, to entertain, to socialize, to bond, to acculturate, and to cope; for comfort, for love, for family, for tradition, and for fun.

Thus, we have a modern day trifecta of abundance:

- An evolutionary physiological drive to eat enough
- Ubiquitous temptation
- The normalization of overeating

Is it any wonder why maintaining a healthy weight is so challenging?

You're Not Broken

Most people come to me for nutritional counseling or coaching with the feeling that there is something wrong with them. Many have been on an emotional roller coaster of diagnoses, saying they believe their thyroid must be off, their metabolism slow, or their genetics insurmountable. They have tried all types of diets; some worked for a while, but nothing seemed to stick or be sustainable, so something must be wrong with them.

What does *not* work is the thinking that there is a magic pill, potion, recipe, or regimen that causes weight loss. What does *not* work is believing that there is a certain food or nutrient you need to eat or avoid to lose or that you need to push harder or do more in your exercise routine.

It's always the food.

We are biological beings, adapted in a beautiful way, harmonious with nature where we eat for survival and store energy for times of scarcity. There are biochemical and neurological pathways set into play to keep us on course for reproduction and survival of the species. Of *course* we are tempted by calories. Food tastes good because we require it, and we benefit from continuing to consume it. We are programmed to seek sustenance. What is unique about today is that now we have access to food in unprecedented ways. Ironically, we have also adapted our thinking to justify why we should simply relent and allow social stimuli to dictate when, what, and why we eat. In other words, it is too hard to say no and go against the tribe in social situations, so we often simply sacrifice our goals to fit in. In fact, we have bounced to the opposite extreme of explaining away our biology to normalize overeating. More than 42 percent of adults and over 18 percent of children were categorized as obese in the United States according to the latest CDC statistics.[1] Globally, more than 1.9 billion adults were overweight in 2016 (650 million of those categorized as obese).[2] Obesity is becoming average. How can that be a compilation of broken humans?

The answer is that it is not. We are simply acting in accordance with what is—our environment and social climate have changed. Our biology has not. Thus, the solution is to recognize the misfit and change our habits and behaviors to serve our goals. We have to be comfortable in the uncomfortable, and, when faced with constant pressure from everyone around us, consistently choose ourselves.

Once You Know, You Can't Unknow

There are myriad ways to accomplish a shift in your relationship with food, and that is why there is mayhem surrounding messaging about the process.

That said, the magic happens as the journey unfolds, and you discover all that is exposed as you face your relationship with food, the environment and socialization surrounding food, and the underlying belief systems that emerge when you remove the barriers to change. This is where the fun, entertainment, sexiness, and pleasure come in; though it is also where you uncover the vulnerability, the deeply embedded triggers and acculturation, and often the pain that has been subconsciously attached to your food choices.

Indeed, this is a deeply personal expedition; one that can be made permanent because once you know the process and how your body responds to this way of eating, you can't unknow. I tell my clients I want them to achieve a "PhD" in their bodies and weight loss and another one in weight maintenance, so the goal is mastery and the wisdom of experiencing it firsthand. Nobody can take away this knowledge. Success is simply a series of small victories. And those successes are made over many moments throughout the day. Every day. You get to choose to serve your purpose. You get to choose again and again and again. You get to choose you now.

This is a journey that continues as a daily practice and ebbs and flows throughout life. *Choose you now* embodies this practice. *Choose you now* means beginning from your heart. It means having the courage to choose according to where your heart is driving you. No matter what. That doing so will ultimately be in alignment for everyone around you because you will be healthier, more peaceful, more joyful, more effective, and more loving. It means going within to make a decision, rather than to others, to the environment, to anything outside of your wisdom. Be you, emanate you, lead from you . . . that is capital *T* Truth.

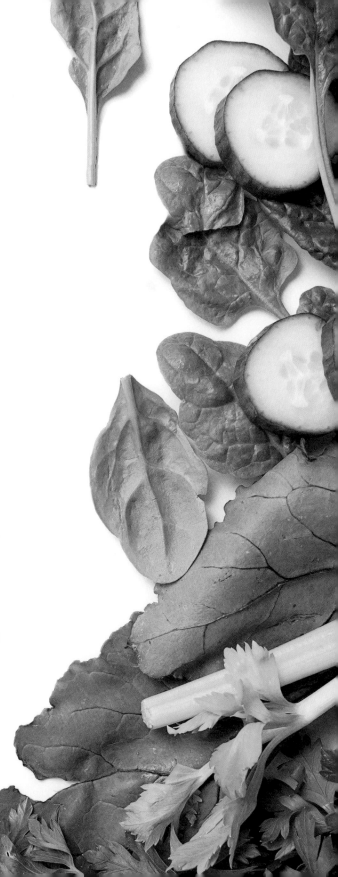

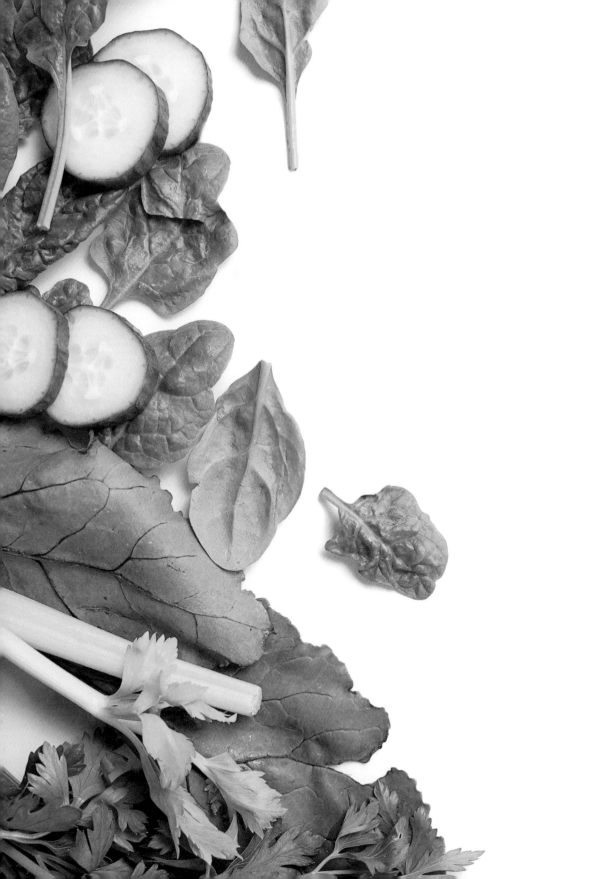

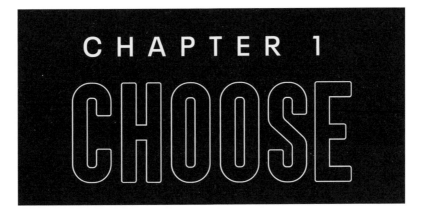

CHAPTER 1
CHOOSE

In my lifelong mission to uncover the secrets to weight loss, I have honed and refined all that I have aggregated with the goal of being able to simplify things. The result is the 10 Tenets to Sustainable Weight Loss–a simplified outline for success. Essentially, these tenets cover everything you need to know about why and how to lose weight for the last time:

1. Find your purpose.

2. Choose your goal weight.

3. Determine your time line.

4. Eat plants. (Whole plants. Nothing but the plants. So help your health.)

5. Learn to recognize hunger and satiety.

6. Don't break the seal.

7. Stop counting.

8. Set a schedule.

9. Monitor meal volume.

10. Master monotony.

I say "simplified," but this does not mean following these tenets is necessarily *easy*. In this chapter and the next, we will dissect and explore these 10 tenets, preparing for the application of the tenets in your everyday life. This chapter is all about what you choose: why you're making this commitment, what you want to achieve, and when you want to do it.

Tenet 1: Find Your Purpose

You can lead a human to healthy, but you can't make them eat. I have personally struggled watching my most beloved ones eat themselves to unhealthy consequences. Even as an expert in the field, writing books and lecturing around the world and on television, I have been painfully unsuccessful at inspiring some of the people closest to me to make a change. Professionally, I am constantly asked how to convince others to change their diet. People reach out to ask if I can help their sister/father/best friend/son/aunt change their diet. After spending years attempting to be persuasive, knowledgeable, and caring enough to change minds, I stopped banging my head against the thick wall of don't-tell-me-what-to-eat innocent people who were minding their own business, quite content with their current diet.

Finally, I relinquished the notion that one can be told how or what to eat and embraced the idea that being a lighthouse is far more effective than being a tugboat. Tactics such as fear, education, guilt, shame, incentivization, and motivation are not the answer–change must come from within. You have to *want* to make a transformation in order to execute and succeed.

This is precisely the inspiration for the title of this book. You have to choose, and you can only choose for yourself.

So, what is your *why*? Why do you want to go through this process? Why have you joined me on this journey in the pages of this book? No matter the reason, it must be something that means a lot to you. Have you or a loved one recently received a concerning diagnosis or experienced a health scare? Do you want to keep up with your children or grandchildren and be a role model for them? Are you simply frustrated with the perpetual cycle of weight loss/weight gain and ready to move on with your life?

It doesn't matter what your "why" is or whether you share it with anyone. All that matters is that you identify your why, shine a light on your why, and apply laser-sharp focus to your why. Write it down. Own it. Decide you will achieve your goals. No matter what.

This is what will drive you to the end. This is the core of determination and persistence. When someone dangles a food that is not on your plan in front of you–a simple truth that will always exist–your why will enable you to choose you.

Tenet 2: Choose Your Goal Weight

You have the power to choose your weight range. There is a clear and simple way to lose weight–create a deficit–and most of us know all too well how to gain weight. Ideal body weight (IBW) is an objective measure calculated by researchers to enable optimal health and create parameters. There is a range of numbers you can use as a reference, and then use that wiggle room to determine what feels the most comfortable for you in your body.

The Hamwi Formula

One of the easiest and most commonly used methods to calculate your IBW is the Hamwi Formula[1]. The Hamwi computations are based on gender, inches, and pounds.

> Male = 106 pounds (48kg) for the first 5 feet (152.4cm) + 6 pounds for each additional inch (1.1kg for each additional cm)
>
> Female = 100 pounds (45kg) for the first 5 feet (152.4cm) + 5 pounds for each additional inch (0.9kg for each additional cm)

For example, the IBW of a 5-foot, 4-inch female is approximately 120 pounds plus or minus 10 percent, depending on the size of the person's frame. So really, this female should aim to weigh somewhere between 108 pounds and 132 pounds. There are online calculators to help, and some science as to why and how this formula is used if you would like to dig deeper.

It is important to note that the Hamwi formula does not account for age, bone density, or fat-to-muscle ratio, all of which impact weight. This segues to this next piece in the formulation.

Size and Shape

Besides the number on the scale, you also need to account for the size of clothing you feel best in and to be aware of the shape of your body. Volume will change with weight loss, but you will likely have the same shape when you reach your goal. You can work on modifying your shape with exercise, but ultimately, the goal is to embrace your natural shape and optimize it for your health and for your level of comfort living in your body.

Even with these tools as references, no one else gets to decide whether or not you need to lose or gain, or whether you are correct in your own assessment. Nobody gets to insult or judge or make decisions for you. This is *your* body. Collect the necessary tools to achieve your most comfortable, healthful self, and then embrace the journey.

Tenet 3: Determine Your Time Line

So many of us *live* on a diet: a continuous cycle of losing and regaining, ups and downs, highs and lows. Let's reframe this so that the goal is to lose weight for the last time. The way to do this is to simply choose it. Decide when you are finally ready (which is probably now since you are reading this), and set aside the necessary time to get to your goal. Do all of your calculations—your IBW and how much weight you have to lose to get there—and allocate about two days per pound (on average) to estimate when you may be done. Whether you have 10, 20, or even 100 pounds to lose, managing your expectations on approximately how long it may take is a helpful data point. If you have a longer way to go, spend some time with the tools for motivation in chapter 4 to reduce the impact of diet fatigue that may set in over time.

Tools for Transformation

First and foremost, there are tools in your armamentarium (my all-time favorite word, defined by Oxford Languages as "a collection of resources available for a certain purpose") to utilize strategically and objectively. Put on your forensics hat, take an unbiased stance, and get ready to study your body and its response to food like never before. The scale isn't sneering up at you, and the amount of weight you have between now and your goal does not in any way make you more or less of your true, beautiful self. You are not broken or less fabulous than you will be at your goal weight. These are data points—facts that can be used to inform your decisions moving forward.

The Scale

Despite the political movement away from using a scale, it is a crucial tool in weight-loss and maintenance success. How else can you check in and stay alert to how your progress is coming other than using a means to measure it? That said, there are a couple of reasons that a scale is less than perfect.

First, most scales cannot accurately discern between water, muscle, body fat, bone, organs, etc. Some scales estimate lean body mass and water, but a consumer scale is not akin to the hydrodensitometry or whole-body air-displacement plethysmography (Bod Pod) scales used in clinical or university settings. Setting aside the fancy terminology, water fluctuations happen, and you will not necessarily know that from your scale. A bit of extra sodium in the day or hormonal waves of fluid retention and release will impact the scale, and it is important to become aware of that. Again, this is information to incorporate as you study your body's responses to food, hormonal shifts, and your biorhythm.

Secondly, intestinal contents can obfuscate (mess with) a weigh-in. With weight loss, there is less food going in—we are creating a deficit—and therefore, there will be less food coming out. (Disclaimer: dietitians love to talk about poop.) Some foods encourage a quicker journey through the gastrointestinal (GI) tract, while others seem to slow down everything. People vary with this detail, and although this is simply anecdotal based on years of working with different people, it is worth noting: it seems as though starchy vegetables (such as potatoes and squash) and soups tend to move more quickly and smoothly through the system, while rice, legumes, and raw salads tend to move a bit slower. There are myriad categories of fibers in these foods, and your microbiome profile adjusts according to your diet, so there are many variables at play here. Take note of which foods work best in your GI tract and which ones are rough. More data points for your journey.

However imperfect, the scale is a baseline and continuous assessment to compare the day-to-day fluctuations. Weigh in daily: first thing in the morning, after voiding, before drinking, and stripped of all clothing and any heavy accoutrements. (I take my hair clip out before stepping on the scale—in the spirit of accuracy.)

Note and monitor the trends, not necessarily the sticky stagnations or minutiae overall. Just monitor and take note. If you go days without losing or you stay at the same weight for too many days, and you know it is not fluid or built-up intestinal contents, it is the food. We will address this throughout the rest of the book.

The Measuring Tape

We do not accurately see ourselves, our *three-dimensional selves.* We see mirrors, photographs, and videos, but it is challenging for most of us to see ourselves in 3D. Similarly, we see what we do see on a daily basis, so it is far more challenging to notice the changes taking place as our weight changes. An example of this is not seeing a niece, nephew, grandchild, etc. for months or years on end and when you do see them, you are blown away by the amount of growth/change that has evolved since last you saw them. Or an actor who has been off the screen for a while who suddenly appears and you can see how much they may have aged (or did not). Distance, time, and space bring clarity.

Thus, as you go through this process, you will not necessarily see the changes. That is where the second tool in your armamentarium (I can't help but enjoy this word at every opportunity)–the measuring tape–comes in handy. It is helpful to maintain a weekly, or even monthly, measurement chart of the circumferences of your biceps, chest, waist, abdomen, hips, thigh, and calf. Measure the same exact place each time, and you will watch your size shift.

Clothing Feels

Another helpful, albeit more subjective, tool to be aware of is how you feel in your clothes. Whether you have been getting on the scale or not, you know how your jeans fit when you put them on fresh from the dryer and try to zip them up. You know when certain clothing items are feeling tighter or looser, and you can use this as yet another data point to assess how things are going. As you begin your journey, note how

many different clothing sizes you have in your closet. No judgment, just awareness. Every few weeks, check in to see which clothes feel the most comfortable, and make a note.

Another motivational tool I suggest to my clients is to choose outfits you cannot wait to fit into–either ones from the past or new teasers you have been eyeing–and make them visible. Either bring them out of hiding or keep a photo handy of one you want to try on in the near future. These little messages can be surprisingly motivating.

Now that you have your why, are ready to begin, and have been armed with some basic tools, let's dig into the details: what to eat, when, and how much, along with some mental hacks and focal points to get you through the rough moments. Again, this is simple but not always easy. It is a journey, and perhaps this is the best–or, at least, the most transformational–part.

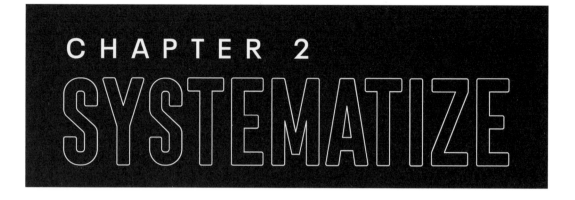

CHAPTER 2
SYSTEMATIZE

I would like to invite you to think about food and diet in a different way, perhaps in a way you haven't prior to now. Think back to our modern day trifecta of abundance from the introduction: the evolutionary drive to consume, the availability of food, and the normalization of overeating. We are deeply socialized to use food for celebration, comfort, connection, entertainment, and relaxation. Instead of merely viewing food as sustenance and nourishment, there are myriad variables that significantly impact our daily lives when it comes to how, what, why, and when we eat.

During this journey, a fundamental part of the transformation–the part that will make this sustainable and permanent–is to think of food objectively and to understand why you eat the way you do. The moments of clarity and awareness that you can identify allow you to make mindful, conscientious decisions moving forward. This chapter is about setting systems into place so that you are in the driver's seat, dictating your progress, accumulating awareness, and moving toward success.

Tenet 4: Eat Plants

Eat plants. Whole Plants. Nothing but the plants. So help your health. Data consistently show that a whole-food, plant-based diet is ideal for weight loss and sustainable weight-loss management.[1,2,3] Myriad factors come into play, including the low caloric density of most plant foods, the increased satiation and satiety due to higher fiber content, and the ability to up the volume a bit more than you can on any other diet. Most importantly, you can lose weight in many different ways; doing so with plants just happens to be the most health-promoting way possible.

Diet is the number-one cause of early death and disability in the world.[4] There are a plethora of health benefits associated with eating plants, including the fact that a plant-based diet is the only diet that has been associated with reversing advanced-stage cardiovascular disease[5,6] and type 2 diabetes.[7,8] Plant-based diets have also been associated with reduced risk of mortality, cardiovascular disease, type 2 diabetes, certain cancers, high blood pressure, high cholesterol, and hyper- glycemia; lower body fat and BMI; and reduced medication requirements.[9,10,11,12,13,14, 15,16,17,18]

In addition to all of these well- substantiated benefits, there are many more studies in the works with optimistic results for kidney disease, gastrointestinal disorders, Alzheimer's, autoimmune diseases, and more. While this is anecdotal, I like to add that I have also seen hundreds of clients in my nutrition practice experience extraordinary (and sometimes unexpected) side effects after switching to a plant-based diet, including overcoming lifelong asthma and eczema; reducing acne, aches, and pains; and more.

What's on the Plate

This begs the question, then, what exactly defines a whole-food, plant-based diet? As with weight loss, we need to simplify plant-based diets, too.

Let's start with what is *not* included in this way of eating, so we can get that out of the way and focus on all the deliciousness that *is* included and emphasized throughout the remainder of this book.

All animal products plus refined oils, sugars, and flours are limited or, ideally, completely eliminated when eating a whole-food, plant-based diet. The fewer of these products consumed, the better. This includes all meat, poultry, seafood, eggs, and dairy. Free range, organic, grass-fed, wild-caught, and/or sustainably farmed versions of all of the above are also excluded in a plant-based diet.

Heavily processed foods need to be avoided as well: products with added sweeteners, oils, flours, salts, preservatives, colorings, flavorings, and other adulterants. This includes many types of bread, sweetened beverages, baked goods, fried foods, breaded foods, crackers, bars, most dried fruits, most commercial dressings and sauces, and almost all restaurant food. Practice focusing on the ingredients list when reading food labels and ignoring everything else on the package to avoid confusion.

Oil is a processed food: pure fat that has been extracted from a whole plant, removing all of the fiber and most of the nutrition. It is nutritionally unnecessary when food is not scarce. It served its purpose during times of scarcity, but now that much of the world has access to unlimited calories, we do not need to seek out maximally caloric-dense options. This is especially relevant when trying to lose weight. Fortunately, with a few tweaks in the kitchen, you can remove oils and—at 120 calories and 14 grams of fat per tablespoon—the result is you can save hundreds or thousands of calories of pure fat from your diet. This means removing all oils, including olive oil, hempseed oil, grapeseed oil, canola oil, and especially coconut oil, which is extra high in saturated fats and has been found to be not much better than butter for your arteries.[19]

Similar to oil, sugar is refined of fiber and nutrition, and there are many negative health consequences associated with its consumption. Generally, the guidelines are to keep added sweeteners to less than 5 percent of total calories. Instead of calculating all of that, you can simply choose to avoid foods and beverages with added sweeteners, including low- or no-calorie sweeteners. You will find recipes in this book that include a bit of maple syrup, molasses, or fruit-based sweeteners to add sweetness and balance to certain recipes. They are used in small enough doses to meet this recommended allowance.

Finally, sodium should be kept to a minimum. According to the American Heart Association, no more than 2,300 milligrams (mg) of sodium a day and an ideal limit of no more than 1,500 mg per day for most adults, especially for those with high blood pressure is advised. They suggest that even cutting back by 1,000 mg a day can improve blood pressure and heart health.[20] This is usually quite simple to do when avoiding heavily processed foods, as this is where sodium is sneaky and omnipresent. If you are used to eating higher levels of salt in your diet, know that your palate will adjust with time and consistency. As you lower your threshold for saltiness, you will begin to notice the natural saltiness in whole foods, and your palate will come alive with enhanced taste acuity.

Of special note are the plethora of plant-based meats, eggs, and dairy that are now ubiquitous in the marketplace. While most of these products are better options than the animal-based versions, be aware that they, too, often contain high amounts of saturated fat (usually from tropical oils, especially coconut and palm oils), sugars, and other compounds that are disease-promoting. While these can be included as a "day-of-deliciousness" treat food once in a while on a health-promoting diet, they should by no means be considered staple foods. The goal is to stick with the "whole-est" foods possible, which are listed in the next section.

This may sound impossible, but navigating this way of eating is like learning a new language. First, you introduce some new ingredients you have not yet tried (like the new alphabet of a foreign language). Then, you learn to string these ingredients into recipes and menus (as the letters become words and sentences) until finally, the recipes and menus are familiar, effortless, and enjoyable (as it is to become fluent in a new language).

We will dig deeper into the practical aspects of applying these guidelines to your meals in chapter 3, with information on ingredients and culinary tips.

But now, as promised, here is the beautiful bright side of what is celebrated, enjoyed, and on-plan in this way of eating—a whole-food, plant-based diet consists of vegetables, fruits, whole grains, legumes, mushrooms, nuts, seeds, herbs, and spices in infinite tasty combinations! When I say infinite, I truly mean there is no limit to creative, tasty ways to mix and match these ingredients and create your new (and a rebranding of your old) favorite foods. If you want to lose weight and optimize your health, eating a diet based on whole plants is at the top of the list.

Change Your Palate

If you are new to this way of eating– especially if you are accustomed to consuming more processed foods–you may discover that your palate needs to adapt. Initially, whole foods may taste a bit bland if you are used to eating foods that are refined into flours, sugars, and oils and/or processed with additives, artificial flavors, and preservatives. Foods that are considered hyperpalatable–usually those with sugars, flours, fats, and salts–elicit neurological and behavioral responses that are similar to those produced by drugs of abuse.[21] They stimulate dopamine releases in the brain that keep you wanting more.

Interestingly and fortunately, however, taste buds are dynamic. Cells within taste buds are continuously turning over such that approximately 10 percent of cells are new to each taste bud each day.[22,23] This means that as you stick with this wholesome way of eating, the food becomes tastier and tastier, and soon, the nuances become amplified. Fruit and a sweet potato begin to taste as sweet as candy. The salt in celery and chard become more pronounced. The natural umami of mushrooms and tomato paste are more noticeable. The mouthfeel and flavor of starch (arguably considered the sixth taste) is satisfying. And the sensory properties of fat (creaminess, oiliness, and thickness) are more overt in foods like nuts, seeds, tofu, and avocado. Have patience with the simplicity of flavors, knowing their taste intricacies and collective synergies will be far more noticeable and appreciated with time.

Find your recipe repertoire. Find the recipes you enjoy that are made from any of the infinite tasty combinations of vegetables, fruits, whole grains, legumes, mushrooms, nuts, seeds, herbs, and spices. You only need to start with one recipe. If you love it, keep it in the rotation. If you do not love it, modify it or move on.

By continuing to eat in this way and refraining from "breaking the seal" with bites and bits of hyperpalatable foods, you will retrain your palate and begin to genuinely enjoy the natural sweet, salty, starchy, umami, and oily characteristics of whole plants.

Avoid Macroconfusion

There are three energy-containing macronutrients found in our food (well, four if you include alcohol): fat, carbohydrate, and protein. While these are biochemistry terms used for classification, they have been misused and misinterpreted in the last several decades, confusing everyone, from people trying to understand what exactly they should eat to researchers trying to distill science and physiology into useful recommendations.

The evidence on an ideal macronutrient profile of a diet for weight loss or for health is inconclusive. There is evidence indicating that a higher-fat diet is healthful, such as the Mediterranean diet, as well as evidence showing that a low-fat diet, such as that studied in Okinawa, Japan, is optimal.[24,25,26,27, 28,29] There are also studies that conclude that both low carbohydrate consumption and high carbohydrate consumption increase mortality risk . . . in the same study![30] How is anyone to make sense of this, let alone make practical decisions based on this conflicting information? The answer is that it is a waste of time, energy, and resources.

Secondly, both a baked potato and a doughnut would be classified by many as a "carb." This is because they both contain carbohydrates–a similar amount of carbohydrates, actually. If you dig deeper, you'll find that the doughnut is almost half fat and half carbohydrate, but the doughnut's carbohydrate is coming predominantly from sugar–31 percent of the doughnut's total calories. This is a giant conundrum if you are trying to tell people to eat fewer carbs or less fat. It is far simpler, clearer, and more accurate to say, "Eat more starchy vegetables and fewer refined baked goods."

Baked Potato (100 grams)
93 calories
2.5g protein (11% of calories)
0.1g fat (<1% of calories)
63.2g total carbohydrate
   2.2g fiber
   17.3g starch
   1.2g sugar

Doughnut (100 grams)
417 calories
4.5g protein (4% of calories)
20g fat (43% of calories)
57.4g total carbohydrate
   2.2g fiber
   0g starch
   32g sugar

These are two fundamental reasons it is far better to eliminate macronutrient-speak–*macroconfusion*–from any nutrition reference and bring the conversation back to foods we all recognize.

Caloric Density

Whole-plant foods–particularly fruits, vegetables, and mushrooms–contain fewer calories per a given weight than many animal products and processed foods. They are high in nutrients and low in calories, meaning you get the most nutritional bang for your caloric buck.

Although this is a helpful principle to keep in mind, it is also not accurate to say that you can eat as much food as you want, whenever you want, if you are eating plants. This is a myth often echoed in weight-loss recommendations that winds up leaving people who listen to that advice feeling frustrated and broken.

Two main problems occur with this philosophy: dietary fatphobia and binge/purge perpetuation.

Dietary Fatphobia

It is easy to see why using caloric density as a primary model by which to lose weight can be tempting. Fat contains 9 kilocalories (kcals) per gram while carbohydrate and protein contain 4 kcals per gram (alcohol contains 7 kcals per gram). Therefore, why not decrease fat consumption and emphasize carbohydrate- and protein-rich foods? With this in mind, there have been movements throughout the decades to

Caloric Density

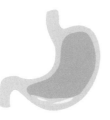

400 calories of oil

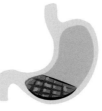

400 calories of beef

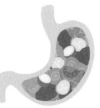

400 calories of vegetables

Stretch receptors are located throughout the stomach. When they are triggered by food, they send signals to your brain to tell you to stop eating. With high-fiber, whole-plant foods, you can eat the most quantity for the least amount of calories.

simply eat less fat. In recent years, there have been ideas thrown around that you can eat as much as you want so long as you avoid fat to the greatest extent possible.

But fat is not bad for you. In fact, we require certain essential fatty acids to come from our diet. While a low-fat, whole-food, plant-based diet has been consistently associated with weight loss and weight-loss maintenance, along with reduction of risk and reversal of advanced cardio-vascular disease, type 2 diabetes, and many other chronic diseases; this does not mean avoiding fat completely is a long-term strategy for success.

When attempting to lose weight rapidly using a very low-calorie diet (VLCD), there is a risk of gallstones. This has been seen in the science using liquid meal replacements that were too low in fat. A study published in 1998 concluded that adequate fat intake

is essential for gallstone prevention.[31] Of course, VLCDs should be done under the supervision of a healthcare provider, but knowing this helps mitigate the risk when focusing on weight loss.

There is an abundance of research showing the advantages of consuming foods like nuts and seeds (1 to 2 ounces or 30 to 40 grams per day) for optimal health and to support weight loss and weight management.[32,33,34,35,36,37,38,39,40] This is why most of the dressings and sauces in the recipes of this book are based on nuts and seeds. You can ideally include a quarter- to half-cup total of nuts and seeds a day to equal the recommended intake. Foods like tofu (and most whole soy products) and avocado are also considered high-fat foods, yet these offer wonderful nutrient profiles and health advantages, too.[41,42,43,44,45,46,47]

Caloric and Nutrient Density of Food Changes with Processing

For the most nutritional bang for your caloric buck and to help with weight loss by enhancing satiety with fewer calories, focus on the most intact forms of food as often as possible.

Minimally Processed ·······> (Intact)	Moderately Processed ·······> (Removes Fiber/Water/Nutrients)	Highly Processed (More Calories, Less Satiety, Fewer Nutrients)
Grapes ·····>	Raisins ·····>	Grape Juice
Wheatberries ·····>	Whole Grain Bread ·····>	White Flour
Olives ·····>	Olive Paste ·····>	Olive Oil
Sugar Beets ·····>	Molasses ·····>	Refined Sugar
Brown Rice ·····>	Brown Rice Pasta ·····>	Rice Flour
Nuts and Seeds ·····>	Nut and Seed Butter ·····>	Nut and Seed Oil

Furthermore, fat in the diet enhances taste and palatability of foods. And many people become so afraid of eating fat that they avoid these healthful, nutritionally dense nuggets.

Therefore, instead of fearing fat and instead of focusing on macros, the recipes in this book are balanced and include a weight loss-supporting dose of healthy fats.

Binge/Purge Perpetuation

A significant, potential problem for sustainable weight loss and maintenance is that calorie-dense foods reinforce overeating. The more you acclimate to the sensation of fullness, as is common in binge eating, the more you seek that sensation. We have stretch receptors in the stomach that detect the distension of the stomach wall in the presence of food, and then directly stimulate signals to the brain to trigger satiation and the reduction of appetite.[48] Regular bouts of stomach distention may exacerbate chronic overeating.[49]

Instead of masking symptoms (overeating) by finding foods we can eat more of and fill our bellies with (i.e., avoiding fat), it is healing and proactive to address the core issue, which is overeating, and often includes the desire to be adequately or excessively full. Thus, the long-term goal is not to see how much food we can eat and still achieve or maintain a healthy weight but rather to address overeating conscientiously, with purpose, and in a way that is maintainable for the long haul. Rediscovering comfortable satiation without challenging the max capacity of the stretch receptors is something worth practicing. Because everything about food is habit, recognizing true hunger and satiation—and then letting that guide your consumption–are key. See Tenet 5 for more on this.

This strategy enables us to eat a well-balanced diet including healthful nuts, seeds, avocados, and soyfoods as well as to habituate to sustainable hunger/satiety regulation.

How to Use Caloric Density

Instead of avoiding fat and aiming to see how much food you can eat and get away with in terms of continuing weight loss, here are four ways to incorporate all of the advantages of this principle into your diet without the risks.

1. **Volumize**: Plump up meals with more veggies, mushrooms, and fruits.

   Nonstarchy vegetables, mushrooms, certain fruits, as well as some starchier foods contain the fewest calories per gram of all foods. You can always add more of these lower-calorie foods so you fill up with less. Preload a more calorically dense meal with a simple salad of mixed greens, tomato, cucumber, fresh herbs, and perhaps a splash of citrus or vinegar; or a cup of vegetable soup.

2. **Maximize:** Make foods with low caloric density the main attraction.

   Use the principle of caloric density by emphasizing lower calorie-dense foods as main ingredients in recipes. For example, foods like cauliflower, mushrooms, spaghetti squash,

eggplant, and butternut squash are very low in calories yet satiating. They also make excellent staple ingredients.

3. **Prioritize:** Minimize foods with high caloric density.

   Higher on the caloric-density scale and not included in the list of whole-plant foods (vegetables, fruits, whole grains, legumes, mushrooms, nuts, seeds, herbs, and spices) are items such as breads and other foods made from flours, meats, and oils.

   Included, but higher in calories, are avocados, whole grains, legumes, nuts, seeds, and nut and seed butters. Prioritize the foods with lower caloric density and minimize these higher-calorie foods. For nutritional and health reasons, be sure to include 1 to 2 ounces (30 to 40 grams or ¼ to ½ cup) of nuts and seeds per day, ideally as a base for a dressing or sauce, and use the other foods sparingly.

4. **Recognize:** Hone in on hunger and satiety.

   Recognize your hunger and satiety signals, and you may even notice how little it takes to reach satiety with fewer calories. We will delve into this in the next section.

Calories of Certain Representative Foods per 100 grams

For reference, here is an array of foods and their calories per equal-sized weights (100 grams). Note that animal products are listed for context.

Food	Kcals/100 g	Food	Kcals/100 g	Food	Kcals/100 g
>50 kcal		Butternut squash (cooked)	40	**>200 kcal**	
Coffee	2	Carrots (raw)	41	Beef tenderloin	218
Herbal tea	2.4	Snap peas	42	Bagel	257
Cucumber	12	Grapefruit	42	Whole-grain bread	265
Iceberg lettuce	14	Beets	43	Dates	282
Celery	16	Brussels sprouts (raw)	43	French/sourdough bread	289
Zucchini (boiled)	16	Kale (raw)	50		
Romaine lettuce	17	Pineapple	50	**>500 kcal**	
Tomato (raw)	18			Pumpkin seeds	541
Green bell pepper	20	**50–100 kcal**		Cashews	553
Zucchini (raw)	21	Apple	52	Almonds	575
Cauliflower (cooked)	23	Mandarin oranges	53	Dark chocolate	578
Spinach (raw or cooked)	23	Shiitake mushrooms (cooked)	56	Tahini	570
Cabbage (cooked)	23	Blueberries	57	Peanut butter	588
Cabbage (raw)	25	Mango	65	Walnuts	654
Cauliflower (raw)	25	Grapes	69	Coconut oil	862
White mushroom (stir-fried)	26	Corn kernels	81	Olive oil	884
Spaghetti squash	27	Kidney beans	84		
Cremini mushrooms (raw)	27	Banana	89		
Brown mushrooms (cooked)	28	Sweet potato (baked)	90		
Kale (cooked)	28	Russet potato (baked)	97		
Watermelon	30				
Jalapeño	30	**>100 kcal**			
Green beans	31	Brown rice	112		
Strawberries	32	Lentil	116		
Cantaloupe	34	Quinoa	120		
Broccoli (raw)	34	Pasta	131		
Broccoli (cooked)	35	Tofu	145		
Grilled portobello	35	Chicken breast	151		
Eggplant	35	Avocado	160		
Brussels sprouts (cooked)	36	Chickpeas	164		
Parsley	36	Soybeans	172		
Jicama	38	Salmon	182		
Onion (raw)	40				

Tenet 5: Learn To Recognize Hunger and Satiety

The most important signals to reacclimate yourself with are hunger and satiety—identifying when you are truly hungry and then satisfied with *just enough*. These are monumentally important tools for the long haul. Despite sounding obvious, these are skills that require practice and patience.

Use a scale of zero to ten, where zero is completely empty and ten is Thanksgiving/holiday-stuffed plus an additional serving of pumpkin pie. Work to eat when you most closely approach zero and stop when you are *just* satiated. This requires quite a lot of practice and intensive mindfulness, but everything about food is habitual, and these skills can be learned and honed. Practice daily with each meal, beginning with each bite. Know that you could technically get away with not eating anything, relying on your stored adipose tissue to fuel your body's needs.

I am not suggesting you fast—in fact, I advise against it during weight loss. Fasting is different from time-restricted feeding in that this usually implies longer periods of time without eating any food. The definition of *fast* is in the eye of the beholder as there are different schools of thought on this. There are long-term water-only fasts, intermittent or alternate-day fasts, periodic fasting, very low-calorie diets, and time-restricted feeding/eating (TRF). While there is abundant evidence supporting extraordinary health benefits of each of these types of fasting, TRF allows the healthy individual to gain the benefits in a civilized, comfortable way that does not have the same type of risks or discomfort that may be associated with the more restrictive types of fasting. Fasting for longer than three to five days should be supervised by a qualified medical professional. Most people can not only survive this mild restriction of calorie, but can thrive with it. A combination of whole-food, plant-based diets with TRF appears to be one of the most ideal ways to eat for long-term weight management and enhanced healthspan and longevity.

The Celery Stick Test

When you are hungry, everything sounds delicious. This is why we overspend or overbuy when we head to the grocery store hungry. Notice that the hungrier you become, the more foods sound and look appealing. However, after you have finished a meal, fewer and fewer foods are tempting. This is also why you may feel that nothing sounds good when trying to plan a menu or look in your pantry for something to eat when you are not eating for hunger. I use the "celery stick test" as a reference, as it is not a food that tempts most people frequently. (If celery never tempts you, try using a fresh, crisp apple for this exercise instead.) If you are hungry enough to be tempted by a celery stick (or an apple), it is likely time to eat.

Can You Stop Now?

Stop eating as soon as you feel the inkling of satiety. Of course, you will want more. We are survivors biologically and many of us–myself for certain–do not have an off switch. It is quite easy to overeat as we have momentum and are enjoying the meal. What's one more bite? Why not simply finish the plate?

Remember that you need to create a deficit to lose weight and this starts right now. Put down your fork or spoon and ask yourself, "What if this is my last bite?" as well as, "Can I be finished and continue with my day?" Even if you may need to return to eating sooner rather than later, try stopping short of what you normally do. It may surprise you how effortless this is once you make the decision.

Whatever you do, don't aim for feeling "full." Pushing past satiation will invariably lead to gain or, at best, a flat line (no loss). Remind yourself how temporary this is, and that this is not supposed to be fun, pleasurable, entertaining, or satisfying. This is weight loss–time for a real deficit. Fill those newfound gaps with nourishing, rewarding, stimulating, and exciting activities, projects, experiences, and gifts. I have clients who are finally finishing their PhD dissertations, knitting sweaters, taking classes, connecting spiritually, relaxing, learning new languages, rekindling or deepening relationships, starting businesses, and so much more–simply because they honored their drive to lose weight and let go of using food for anything other than nourishment for a temporary, finite period of time. Your world expands and life enhances when you allow yourself to let go of food as anything other than sustenance.

Tenet 6: Don't Break The Seal

Many people find that all it takes is one bite to fall off their plan. One bite of something hyperpalatable leads to a downward spiral that is difficult to stop. Examples I often hear include a single french fry, a piece of bread from the bread basket, a slice of pizza, one chip, a bite of cake, a piece of candy. That first bite lights up the brain and leaves you wanting more. All too often, it is never enough. You will likely never be satisfied. And this is why we overeat or binge on certain foods. It is a natural biochemical response. That is what happens when you tempt your taste buds and your resolve.

How could you not go all in once you have that explosion of flavor and burst of feel-good hormones our brain releases into our bloodstream? You are human, after all.

But if you prioritize yourself, reaching your goal on purpose, aiming to support your why, none of that momentary deliciousness can distract you. Nothing in the moment tastes as good as healthy and lean feels long term. Nothing. Stay on-plan. Don't break the seal.

Tenet 7: Stop Counting

While I shared the calorie content of different foods in the section on caloric density, this was only for illustration and by no means encouragement to count what you consume. Calories, grams, macros, blah blah blah. I may be the only dietitian who doesn't track, but that is because counting is a black hole of confusion and frustration. This program is instead about turning within, fulfilling your deep desires, and achieving mastery. Go within. Practice mindfulness. You know your body or if you don't quite yet, you certainly will by the end of this process. If you stick to a diet of vegetables, fruits, whole grains, legumes, mushrooms, nuts, seeds, herbs, and spices and follow the 10 Tenets, you will lose weight and achieve optimal health—at the same time. It's the ultimate win-win.

Tenet 8: Set a Schedule

Giving yourself time off from the fed state is a gift to your cells. Time-restricted eating (also known as *time-restricted feeding*) is associated with reductions in weight, fat mass, waist circumference, triglycerides, blood pressure, inflammatory markers, and improvements in blood cholesterol, metabolic parameters, blood sugar regulation, and much more. The research continues to build in support of eating within a shortened time frame each day as opposed to staying in the fed state.[50,51,52,53]

Let your miraculous body do its job—all the metabolic housecleaning it requires to thrive. You do not need to eat continuously throughout the day. No need to "stoke the metabolism," "manage your energy levels," or "avoid hunger." That is all marketing and obfuscation.

After the last bite of food, it takes four to six hours for your body to digest and absorb, and there is a whole cascade of hormones that are released and physical mechanisms that have to occur. This is a very labor-intensive process, diverting blood and energy from everywhere else in the body toward the GI tract.[54] If you are

constantly in the fed state, the body does not have the need to tap into its fat storage. It also inhibits autophagy, which translates to "self-eating," and is a healthy stressor on the body that occurs with nutrient deficit and is necessary to support healthy metabolic housekeeping.[55]

Eat less frequently—within a shortened window. Most of my clients stick to a four- to six-hour window, but some stay within eight hours. Find what works best for you, and contain eating within that time frame. Manage that by avoiding breaking the seal with snacks or a bite of this or that. You can drink calorie-free beverages during this time, including water, sparkling water, coffee, espresso, and tea (black, oolong, white, green, or herbal). Your body will acclimate to this schedule over time, especially if you stick to eating at the same time(s) each day. Our circadian clocks are brilliant, and everything about food is habit. You can adjust and grow comfortable with new habits.

Eat on purpose. Once or twice a day is fine. You must create a deficit to lose weight. Optimizing nutrition comes later.

Tenet 9: Monitor Meal Volume

This is perhaps the trickiest part. "How much do I need to eat?" is the question I get most frequently, and I do not have a specific answer. This is where interindividual variability comes into play. Fortunately, we have both objective and subjective tools to utilize conscientiously. If the scale does not go down and you are only eating within that four- to six-hour window, you are simply eating too much volume.

Use the scale, but remember that fluid shifts (due to hormones or sodium, most commonly) and temporary constipation (which is all too common when you are putting less food through the system) impact the scale. Natural fluctuations are common. Focus on the trend. Watch the curves and practice radical self-compassion when those bumps up don't reflect your consistency and determination. Stay the course; you are losing body fat every day if you are not eating too much. Overeating is the most common cause of stagnation, so in that case, simply eat less the next day.

Tenet 10. Master Monotony

This fantastic quote is attributed to motivational speaker Zig Ziglar: "Repetition is the mother of learning, the father of action, which makes it the architect of accomplishment." And we have always heard that "practice makes perfect." When it comes to food, the idea of repetition versus variety is crucial.

Greater dietary variety has been found in the research to increase consumption and body weight, as well as body fat. Research demonstrates that reducing food group variety can be implemented and does reduce energy (calorie) intake in the diet.[56] Furthermore, it has been found that limiting variety can help with successful weight-loss maintenance.[57]

The fewer decisions you have about meals/eating/recipes, the easier and quicker this will go. Experiment with different types of recipes to determine which you enjoy eating, keep you satiated, cause the least disruption in your GI tract, and are manageable to prepare. I've found that soups tend to be easiest for most people. Experiment with tweaking a small sampling of recipes, and you will find your favorites. You can stick to one or two recipes for weeks at a time safely. Remember: this is about deficit, not optimal nutrition. This is temporary. Make it as simple as possible so you get this part done. Once and for all.

You've Got This

This is all you need to reach your weight-loss goals—literally all you need to know about losing weight. You may think this sounds overly simple and, alas, it really is.

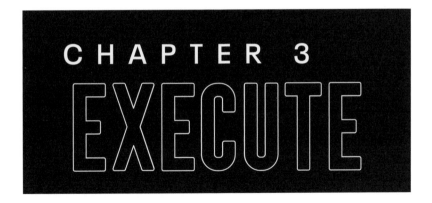

CHAPTER 3

EXECUTE

Now that you have all of the tools and concepts to get started, you can apply them using the delicious, nutritious, balanced recipes in the chapters ahead. Here is how to utilize this information as simply and methodically as possible.

Meal Planning: Plan, Experiment, Adjust

Give a person a meal plan, and you feed them for a day. Teach a person how to plan meals, and you feed them for a lifetime.

Most people try to hire me to create a meal plan for them. Many simply want to know exactly what they need to eat to lose weight. However, I refuse to make meal plans because what happens after you finish following them for a while? You do not have the confidence, wisdom, and wherewithal to make future food decisions.

My goal with my clients and with you, my reader, is to empower you to achieve a PhD in your body during weight loss and once

again with weight maintenance. By the end of this journey, you will know exactly what, when, and how much you need to eat to lose. While we are mostly all the same genetically and even physiologically, there are some minor interindividual variations with certain things like taste preference, environment, gastrointestinal (GI) tolerance and bowel movement habits, social pressures, and emotional reactions to food.

The key is to analyze, assess, and accommodate. In order to achieve a PhD, you must study, focus, learn, and evolve the experience. Do whatever you need to do in order to understand as much as you can about the day-to-day experiences and overall trends. Document what you eat, when you eat, how your bowels feel and move, how your GI tract responds to each recipe or type of food, and which recipes are most satiating. Assess your progress by getting on the scale every morning, measuring your circumference every couple of weeks, and taking tons and tons of notes. Adjust accordingly.

Putting It All Together

In the spirit of simplicity, which is the antidote to all the mythology and confusing messages everywhere, this is the basic overall plan:

1. **Eat within a time-restricted window,** ideally four to six hours. Try to maintain the same schedule each day.

2. **Choose and make a recipe or two from this book.** Stick with just those one to two recipes for a few days. Notice how each recipe feels, satiates, and moves through you.

3. **Get on the scale every morning and track the results.** Use a food journal to document the date, your weight, time eaten, recipe eaten, approximately how much was eaten (using your fist as an estimate for 1 cup), and anything notable (e.g., bloating, constipation, a meal that was extra satisfying, etc.).

When the scale continues to trend down, repeat. If the scale is stubborn, and it isn't for one of the reasons listed on the next page, eat less or switch recipes.

Begin your approach to the Choose You Now Diet by perusing the recipes here in this book and select one or two that seem easy, that use ingredients you already have (or mostly have) at home, and that look like they fit your palate. Make the recipe and eat it when you are truly hungry. Eat only enough until you are satisfied. Then take notes.

The goal is to experiment with different types of recipes and find your weight-loss recipe repertoire. Identify the recipes that are the most satisfying, that you enjoy eating, that cause the least disruption to your GI tract, and are easy (or at least manageable) to prepare.

Noteworthy trends I have noticed with clients over the years—these observations are anecdotal, not scientific—are . . .

- Most people thrive with soups.
- Salads and whole grains (especially rice) tend to be more constipating than starchy veggies and soups.
- Certain recipes tend to feel best for people and become the staple, go-to choices throughout this process.
- The fewer components to a meal, the easier it is. This is why sticking to one or two recipes at a time is so helpful.

Experiment with tweaking a small sampling of recipes, and you will find your favorites. You can stick to one or two recipes for weeks at a time safely.

The guidelines for using caloric density apply across the board for the totality of the diet.

- Volumize: plump up meals with more veggies, mushrooms, and fruits.
- Maximize: make low-calorie foods the main attraction.
- Prioritize: minimize high-calorie foods.
- Recognize: hone in on hunger and satiety.

When The Scale Doesn't Go Down

There are really only three reasons the scale stalls during weight loss or does not trend down: too much food being consumed, water fluctuations, or a buildup of intestinal contents.

Shift happens. Fluid shifts and intestinal contents move at different paces, depending on hormones, sodium intake (sodium is hidden everywhere), types of foods consumed, liquid consumed, and more. The key is to watch the trends. If, after several days of eating on-plan, you don't see the scale trending down, examine what you are eating and try a different recipe, and/or hone in on the three controllable variables: meal frequency, meal volume, and meal monotony.

Modify accordingly and continue to monitor. Remember that you are not broken; it is always the food.

Noteworthy Culinary Techniques and Ingredients

For those of you who are new to whole-food, plant-based cooking, I want to highlight a few unique strategies and ingredients that may be unfamiliar to help as you navigate this new world. You will notice these sprinkled throughout the recipes; here are some notes to help clarify why they are utilized.

Dry Sautéing

Since we are avoiding oils, it is necessary to be mindful when sautéing to avoid burning and sticking. A nonstick pan can help; however, keep in mind that plastics, many metals (like aluminum), and nonstick coatings can release toxins into your food as it cooks. Choose one of the newer "green" nonstick pans; or consider cast iron, enamel, or stainless steel as safe and functional options. Now, for the technique:

1. Begin by heating the pot or pan. Make sure it is heated through before adding ingredients–when you do add ingredients, they should sizzle.

2. Stay by your pot or pan while you are sautéing because burning can happen quickly. Keep a liquid at arm's reach– usually water or broth–that you can add in slowly.

3. Add the first ingredient to the pan– often this is onion–and let it cook. As it begins to brown, add a bit of liquid (1 tablespoon at a time), stir, watch, and repeat until the ingredient you are cooking has browned or caramelized. (You may need to reduce the heat to brown without burning.)

4. If cooking mushrooms, they will sweat after a few moments. Spread the mushrooms flat on the surface of the pan, without crowding, and let them cook until the liquid is released. After a few minutes, you can stir them and add flavoring, such as tamari, and proceed with the recipe.

Tamari

Tamari is an amazing ingredient that you will see used frequently in this book. Similar to soy sauce, it provides a salty flavor along with umami and balances out recipes really nicely. You can vary this option interchangeably with a gluten-free version, liquid aminos, or soy sauce, and aim for the lowest-sodium version you can find, usually labeled "reduced-sodium." Pay attention to the serving size when comparing brands.

Plant Milk

For the first time in history, supermarkets and coffee shops offer a wall o' plant-based milks. Gone are the days of soy milk or rice milk as the only options. Now there is a plethora of choices—soy, rice, hemp, almond, cashew, and more. While they differ nutritionally and culinarily, opt for whichever variety you prefer (except for coconut milk), make sure it is unsweetened, and be cautious about added flavors if you are using it for a savory application.

Raw Cashews

Cashews are commonly used in plant-based cooking, as they make a wonderful base for creamy sauces and dressings. Raw and unsalted is ideal to avoid excessive sodium. For anyone with an allergy to nuts, hemp seeds make a wonderful, nutritious cup-for-cup replacement.

Worcestershire Sauce

When a recipe calls for Worcestershire sauce, note that it traditionally has anchovies in the ingredients. There are a number of anchovy-free, plant-based options available, which are easy to find.

Sriracha, Hot Sauce, and Ketchup

While offering so much flavor to recipes, these condiments are often high in sodium and sugar. There are some lower-sodium and lower-salt options, but often you will need to order those online, as they are a bit more challenging to find. Note that because these are harder to find, they are used in smaller quantities in these recipes.

Vegetable Broth

Broths are optimally low sodium and one of my favorite options is low-sodium no-chicken broth, which is available online to order if you cannot find it at the store. Or you can opt to make your own simple broth at home to save on cost. Choose your favorite vegetables and seasonings, and make it free of sodium. My favorite method is to combine in a large stockpot 4 cups roughly chopped yellow onion, 2 cups roughly chopped carrots, 2 cups roughly chopped celery, ½ cup sliced shiitake mushrooms, 3 bay leaves, 1 teaspoon black peppercorns, and 10 cups water and simmer for about 45 minutes. Strain out the solids, and store the broth in large Mason jars in the refrigerator for up to 1 week or in the freezer for 4 to 6 months.

Exercise

Contrary to popular belief, exercise slows or disrupts weight loss. While lifelong exercise is fundamental for every organ system, for optimal health and fitness, to slow down aging, to maintain cognitive function, and much more; it also increases appetite and slows down the weight-loss process. Physical activity and exercise is crucial for long-term weight management, so we will bring it back when you transition from weight loss to maintenance mode. In fact, that is precisely how I advise initiating that transition. But for now, take a break from your exercise program. Rest, recover, repair, eat less, binge watch television shows and movies, read books, learn languages, study new skills, meditate, sleep, or whatever else you want to do. Take advantage of this rare opportunity when it is advised you take a break.

You may find that you miss exercise more than you may ever have thought possible, and you will finally be able to separate exercise from weight loss, enabling you to explore all the myriad other reasons to fall in love with moving.

Supplements

Generally speaking, during the weight-loss phase, you can supplement with a multivitamin to cover all the bases. Find one that contains vitamins B12, D, and K2, and the minerals iodine and zinc, so you can release concerns of micronutrient deficiency during this finite period of restriction. You may also consider a microalgae-based, long-chain omega-3 fatty-acid supplement with both EPA and DHA. As always, please ask your healthcare provider to monitor your bloodwork and to supplement according to your personal requirements.

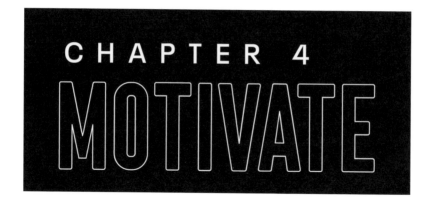

CHAPTER 4
MOTIVATE

Now that you have the theories, tools, and plans in place, it is time to put them into action and stay the course. Struggling to eat healthfully or lose weight is not an information problem. Rather, it is a challenge of staying motivated.

Toolbox for Staying The Course

Essentially, this is the time to use any and all forces to get you to the end. Here are some handy, helpful tools to add to your armamentarium and to give it your all.

Food Journal

Do you remember right now what you ate yesterday? Most people do not remember these details readily. This is one reason food journals are such an important exercise. Documenting what, when, and how much you ate in an ongoing journal offers yet another data point for you. It is an exercise in self-monitoring and a tool to refer back to when you want to identify what exactly works best for you.

Keep it simple so it does not become an overwhelming task. Use an ongoing document on your computer, on your phone, or on paper to jot down the details of your day. I have my clients write down the date and their weight as well as any exercise they did, any beverages they consumed, what time they ate, what their meals consisted of, and an estimate of how much was consumed. (To estimate quantities, a cup is a portion about the size of a fist, and a tablespoon is a portion about the size of a thumb.) I also have my clients include any symptoms they are trying to assess, such as bloating, constipation, or skin reactions, to determine how eating habits may be associated with their specific issues. Collecting this information is exceptionally useful for many purposes.

Perhaps the best benefit of maintaining a food journal is that the exercise of writing itself—simply writing it all down—encourages people to stay on-plan. If you have to write it down and then see it written on the page, it will most likely influence your decisions.

Emotion To-Do Lists

During weight loss, it is important to identify any and all emotions that trigger/ inspire/motivate you to eat when you aren't hungry. There are no reasons to eat other than for nourishment during this time. Now, many of us know this to be true, as it is reasonable. But we are socialized far, far away from this premise.

For example, did your mom, dad, or loved one take you for ice cream or doughnuts when you had a rough day? Did your loved one make you finish your plate so you can earn dessert? Did you meet your friends out for pizza or other comfort food after a break up? Did you ever talk yourself into eating something you knew was unhealthy because it would help you get through something?

What are the main emotions that drive you to eat off-plan? Most commonly, they are stress, boredom, fatigue, or sadness. Eating in celebration is usually due to social pressure and the environment, or perhaps the emotional tug of wanting to be part of the tribe. This emotion list is meant to identify those times you decide to eat off-plan for reasons that are intiated by your feelings. Most of the time, these are unconscious or subconscious decisions, so it may take time to begin to recognize just what is driving you. The way to do this is to stop yourself before your first bite–or, better yet, before you hunt for or prepare food–and ask yourself what you are feeling in that moment. Are you hungry enough to eat a stick of celery or an apple? If not, what exactly is going on in your mind?

Once you have identified any and all of these emotions, begin another list–a separate list for each individual emotion. If you eat to address stress, write a list of any and all activities you can do to relax and calm down–anything you have done or would like to do to soothe yourself that is not food related. If the emotion is boredom, write a separate list of activities that are fun, exciting, and nourishing for your mind and soul. For feeling tired, write a list of restful activities. (Sleep is usually the best one here, but other things like meditation or bathing may help encourage rest.) If it is sadness, what can you do to cheer yourself up or delve into the sadness so you can move through it and work toward catharsis? Whether it is calling a dear friend, listening to music, cuddling your companion animal, or taking a walk in nature; write it down.

These lists should be accessible, ongoing, and exhaustive. Keep adding to them each time you think of something else.

When you find yourself about to eat for any of these reasons, take one minute– set a timer if you need to–and go within. Ask first what is going on, and then bring out the appropriate list. Pick anything on the list and opt for that activity first–before a single bite, before breaking the seal. This may sound mundane or trivial, but these moments are when long-term progress is made. Making these conscious choices may very well be all you need to succeed long term.

Sticky Notes

Many of my successful clients write down reminders on sticky notes and post them on their computers, refrigerators, closets, and cars. Anywhere they want a reminder of their why, they keep these motivational notes and refer to them throughout the day. Here are some of the one-liners we have used:

- Nothing tastes as good as healthy and lean feels.
- Success is a sequential series of small victories.
- Don't break the seal.
- Exercise my "off" switch.
- If not now, when?
- One choice closer to [*fill in the goal*].
- Everything happens in this moment.

It All Happens in This Moment

No matter what your intentions are, no matter how powerful your why, despite all the forethought, everything happens in this very moment. Right now. Each and every decision–to not break the seal, to say no to a temptation, to stay on plan, to eat at the appropriate time and hunger level, to stop when you feel *just* satisfied enough, to eat only foods on-plan–is the single key to your long-term success. Remember that success is a series of small victories, and the only thing you can control is that very moment. Everything happens in these individual moments; don't leave it up to good intentions, hope, and little miracles.

Prepare in Advance

We do not live in a vacuum. There are temptations and opportunities everywhere, all the time: a family member asks you to join them in an indulgence; a friend jokes, "but you haven't had anything fun for weeks"; a colleague invites you to join her for a celebratory piece of birthday cake. These events occur consistently, throughout the year, every year. They are no longer "special treats" reserved for birthdays, anniversaries, and holidays.

The only way to get to your goal is to avoid each and every one of these seductions for a period of time. Until you have found your momentum and are able to attain and sustain your goal, it is optimal to carve out a calculated stretch of weeks, depending on how much weight you want to lose, and avoid these opportunities.

If you can't avoid these situations, prepare for them by knowing exactly what to expect before you go in. If you're going to someone's home or event, inquire about what will be served. If you will be at a restaurant or venue, search ahead of time online or call to see whether you will have options available to you. Having people at your home is easiest, as you will have full control of your meals.

No matter what, there are three main ways to handle being out in the world without full control over the table:

1. **Request options.** You can request options that meet your plan, but this is risky because there is no way to completely control a meal when you are not the one preparing it.

2. **BYOF.** Bring your own food so you know exactly what you are consuming.

3. **Eat ahead of time.** Celebrate the event with the company, conversation, and everything else that is not food. If you are satisfied, it will be easier to say no to food that is off your plan.

If you are uncomfortable facing these challenges at first, wait until you have momentum going and you become more solid. At some point, however, you will likely have to face these types of situations. Steel yourself with a plan in place and, like everything else in life, these experiences will become easier with practice.

Time and Space Heal Everything

Weight loss is essentially a waiting game. Only time can enable the space for your body to use body fat. Unfortunately, we cannot expedite the process, making it go faster than physiology allows.

Remind yourself that time passes, this period is temporary, and the process will end. This is true both in the microcosmic as well as the macrocosmic sense. For example, when you are sitting at a table with a loved one and they are eating something that looks and smells delicious, but is not on your plan, it may be incredibly challenging to not indulge. Your loved one may even offer you a bite or a piece, which

makes it even more challenging. Take note, however, that the intense craving you're experiencing will subside within a few moments . . . as does the food itself when it is no longer available or no longer has the appeal. In situations like these, every single time you say no and stay on-plan strengthens your resolve and gets you closer to the end. The same is true over the long haul as well.

Battling Diet Fatigue

Diet fatigue is real. If you start with 30, 40, 50, or 100 pounds of weight you want to lose, this process can take two, three, four, and up to seven or more months to complete. Surely during this period, special occasions will occur, stress will knock on the door, and holidays will be celebrated. It is a whole lot of saying no, and restriction during temptation after temptation. It is a whole lot of feeling left out of the tribe, isolated, and nonparticipatory. These feelings are real and intense, and they can be exhausting, depressing, and miserable. So how do you stay the course and get to the finish line?

It always comes back to your why. Remind yourself in every way possible—journal, make lists, leave yourself sticky notes everywhere—about why you want this and how good you feel when you stay on-plan.

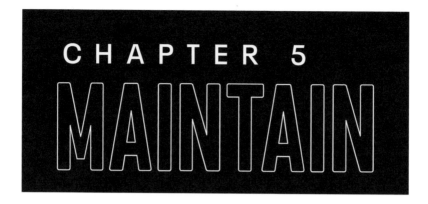

CHAPTER 5
MAINTAIN

Now that you have achieved your goal, the real challenge begins. You may have lost weight before. You may have lost weight more than one time before in your life. In fact, you may relate to the fact that half of Americans try to lose weight each year.[1] Unfortunately, as many of you may have experienced firsthand (I certainly have), the magnitude of realistic, long-term weight loss is significantly lower than what we would hope for and expect.[2] But just like with losing weight, there are strategies to apply for maintenance to ensure that this is the last time you must lose this weight.

Maintenance Mode

The day you see your goal weight appear on the scale is when your new lifestyle begins. It is a sensitive, special time, and you will need to switch your focus from aiming to have the scale move down to keeping that same number on the scale for several days in a row. Keep doing what you have been doing, and use the scale to monitor. The transition needs to be subtle, slow, and conscientious.

Resist the Return to Old Habits

When you reach your goal weight, it is akin to being a spring stretched to max capacity. It will be very easy to catapult back into old habits, prior appetites, and survival mode, thereby undoing what you have successfully accomplished. Avoid letting yourself bounce back. *This* is the key to avoiding that roller coaster ride we are all way too familiar with. *This* is the most important moment.

Fortunately, once again, you have the choice. You have a choice on what to eat, how frequently to eat, how much to eat, and how you adjust your lifestyle over the long run.

Set Boundaries

The first thing to do after reaching your goal is to establish specific boundaries moving forward. Of course, you can't go back to how you were eating before beginning this journey because you will end up where you were going before. And you don't want to go through the weight-loss process again. Research on people who have successfully maintained weight loss over a long period of time indicates that planning ahead, some degree of restriction, self-monitoring, and physical activity are the most important strategies.[3,4]

Here are some suggested boundaries you can set for long-term success and sustainability:

- **Continue to get on the scale every day.** No matter what. Putting off weighing in until Monday, or next week, or sometime in the future will disable your ability to maintain awareness and the data that remind you how to stay on track. Consistent self-weighing is one of the established methods to "help individuals maintain their successful weight loss by allowing them to catch weight gains before they escalate and make behavior changes to prevent additional weight gain."[5]

- **Stick to a defined meal frequency and window of eating.** Routine and habit are helpful for consistency, and your body adjusts to the daily patterns. If you have felt great and achieved your goal weight by eating two times per day within a six-hour window, it will be helpful to stick to this schedule.

- **Maintain a diet based on whole-plant foods.** Making vegetables, fruits, whole grains, legumes, mushrooms, nuts, seeds, herbs, and spices the foundation of your diet will help you maintain your weight loss, as well as offer a reduction in risk of many chronic diseases.

- **Follow the rule of 50 percent.** Make half of every meal fruits and vegetables.

- **Cook at home.** Save dining out for special occasions.

- **Use your tools.** Keep using some or all of the tools from chapter 4, such as your food journal and emotion to-do lists, as well as a gratitude list (see page 49) to self monitor and stay mindful.

Bring Back Movement

Bringing back movement and gentle exercise conscientiously and with purpose is how I transition my clients into maintenance mode. Most people are begging to return to exercise by this point, and it is a great way to start increasing appetite slowly. The key is to tiptoe in with a bit of movement, such as a moderate 30-minute walk, some yoga poses, or light weight lifting. Do it just three or four times a week, and watch the scale. Naturally, your appetite will increase, so let your increased appetite guide you rather than the other way around. If you eat preemptively–eating because you feel you will need more calories to fuel or recover from your workout–you will gain quickly. Let your body use its inner wisdom and continue to eat when hungry and stop when satisfied. If the scale creeps up, rein it in. Slow down.

Physical activity and exercise are crucial predictors of weight-loss maintenance, as well as being crucial for long-term health. Those who successfully maintain weight loss tend to exercise regularly and incorporate movement throughout their day.[6,7] Build back slowly to where you are active each day, targeting each aspect of fitness–endurance, strength, flexibility, balance, and agility. Instead of working out for weight loss–as so many of my clients (and I) had been doing for part of, or even most of, their lives–become mindful here, too. Choose activities you enjoy, that feel great to your body, that inspire you, and keep you feeling energetic, mentally clear, and healthy. Structure your fitness plan accordingly so you can sustain it, and amend it over time.

Introduce Variety

Now that you have become a bona fide creature of habit, it's time to shake things up a bit and start exploring. Maintaining both weight loss and a healthy, well-balanced, whole-food, plant-based diet necessitates some variety in meals. This does not mean, however, that you need to eat something different every day. Most people stick to the same foods in general, but here is where you can aim to optimize your nutrition now that you are done creating and maintaining a deficit.

The 6 Daily 3's

While the simplest way to think about a healthy long-term nutrition plan is to eat a diet based on vegetables, fruits, whole grains, legumes, mushrooms, nuts, seeds, herbs, and spices in infinite tasty combinations, the 6 daily 3's mnemonic can help prioritize your plate for optimal nutrition.

Each of these food groups–cruciferous and leafy green vegetables, other colorful vegetables, fruits, nuts and seeds, legumes, and mushrooms–offers unique nutritional and health advantages. Try to make these the cornerstone for your daily consumption as you plan meals moving forward. (Note that the recipes in this book have this covered.)

Cruciferous and Leafy Green Vegetables

Cruciferous and leafy green vegetables are extraordinary and, if you had to choose, likely the most health-promoting food group, as they offer the most nutritional bang for your caloric buck.

Cruciferae include broccoli, Chinese broccoli, broccoli rabe, Brussels sprouts, cauliflower, kale, collard greens, bok choy, cabbage, kohlrabi, mustard, turnip, radish, watercress, wasabi, daikon, and arugula. In the leafy green category are many of the aforementioned cruciferous choices, as well as lettuces, beet greens, spinach, sea vegetables, and fresh herbs.

Collectively, these gems contain ample fiber, amino acids, and essential fatty acids; and they are exceptionally high in folate, vitamins C, E, and K1 (phylloquinone); the minerals calcium, magnesium, iron, potassium, phosphorus, and zinc; as well as phytonutrients such as chlorophyll (which is the source of their green pigment), provitamin-A carotenoids (typically red, orange, and yellow in pigment, but masked by the dominating green), flavonoids, anthocyanins, coumarins, terpenes, phytosterols, and more.[8]

The 6 Daily 3's

A health-promoting lifestyle begins with these few goals for you and your plate. Aim for just three servings of these six recommended choices every day to reduce your risk for chronic disease and to optimize your overall well-being.

3 servings of cruciferous and leafy green vegetables

1 serving = 1 cup raw or ½ cup cooked and includes: broccoli, kale, cauliflower, Brussels sprouts, lettuce, cabbage, bok choy, sea vegetables, and watercress.

3 servings of fruits

1 serving = 1 medium piece or 1 cup.

3 servings of legumes

1 serving = ½ cup of any bean, hummus, lentil, pea, or soy foods.

3 servings of other colored vegetables

1 serving = ½ cup. Include vegetables from the entire rainbow spectrum, e.g., white-cauliflower, red-beets, orange-carrots, yellow-corn, blue/purple-eggplant, etc.

3 servings of nuts or seeds

1 serving = 1 tablespoon of seeds or ½ ounce (15g) of nuts.

3 servings of mushrooms

Enjoy a minimum of 18 grams of cooked mushrooms per day, or 126 grams per week, or 42 grams 3 times per week (1 cup = 156g). Include at least three different varieties over the week, such as shiitake, oyster, maitake, cremini, portobello, porcini, and enoki.

Cruciferous vegetable consumption protects against cardiovascular disease, metabolic disorders, obesity, diabetes, and cancers, and it offers antimicrobial and anti-aging activities, and more. Their benefits come partly because they contain a potent antioxidant, anti-inflammatory compound called *sulforaphane*.[9,10] When cruciferous vegetables are cut, chopped, or chewed, the enzyme *myrosinase* converts these compounds into the active anticancer form, isothiocyanates. Myrosinase is deactivated by heat, so try chopping the greens and allowing them to sit for a few minutes to allow the reaction to take place before cooking. A healthy hack is to add mustard powder, wasabi, or daikon radish to cooked cruciferous vegetables to initiate this reaction, since they contain myrosinase.

Note that there are compounds called *oxalates* found in many green leaves (as well as other plant foods, such as beets, rhubarb, and amaranth). Oxalates can potentially promote kidney stones and also can inhibit absorption of minerals, such as calcium and iron.[11,12] Therefore, it is best to emphasize the lower oxalate options, namely, cabbage, lettuce, arugula, broccoli, and kale and to minimize the higher oxalate greens, especially spinach, chard, and beet greens.

Enjoy at least three servings a day of these foods, where one serving is equal to 1 cup raw or ½ cup cooked. You will notice a broad array of uses throughout the recipes in this book. You can also increase them in your diet by enjoying the recipes on a bed of raw or cooked greens, or cauliflower or broccoli rice; preloading a meal with a simple green salad or vegetable soup; or by using additional fresh herbs over dishes.

Other Colorful Vegetables

Even though the cruciferous and leafy green vegetables are nutritional rock stars, other colorful vegetables contain concentrated doses of distinctive nutrients that are worthy inclusion in the 6 daily 3's.

- Red, orange, and yellow vegetables—such as bell peppers, sweet potatoes, and squash—are pigmented by carotenoids, powerful phytonutrients, and provitamin A precursors. They support development, growth, immune function, and vision. A majority of the carotenoids in the human diet include beta-carotene, alpha-carotene, lycopene, lutein and cryptoxanthin. They act as powerful antioxidants; protect skin and eyes; and offer cardioprotective, anti-inflammatory, antimutagenic, and anticarcinogenic activities.[13,14]

- White, beige, yellow, and copper colors are found in the *allium* family of vegetables and include garlic, onion, shallot, leeks, and chives. Their main bioactive constituents include organosulfur compounds, polyphenols, and fiber, which confer antimicrobial, antihypertensive, anti-inflammatory, antioxidant, hypolipidemic, antidiabetic, cardioprotective, neuroprotective, antithrombotic, and anticancer activities.[15,16] Include both raw and cooked versions of these foods to maximize their benefits, and consider crushing or cutting garlic and waiting about 10 minutes before consuming so the enzyme *alliinase* can convert alliin to allicin.[17,18]

- Blue, purple, and deep red shades found in vegetables like eggplant, cabbage, beets, purple potatoes, and purple corn are rich sources of *anthocyanins*, polyphenols associated with attenuating obesity and obesity-related inflammation; improving gut microbial health; and reducing risk for cardiovascular disease, cancers, diabetes, some metabolic diseases, and microbial infections. These compounds also improve visual ability and have neuroprotective effects. [19,20,21,22]

Of course, there are other vegetables that offer additional beneficial nutrient compositions, such as celery, parsnips, artichokes, white potatoes, yams, and radishes that may not have an honorable mention but have a lot to offer, nonetheless. Include at least three ½ cup servings of this broad and colorful array of vegetables each day to widen your intake of these crucial compounds.

Fruits

Fruits fall into their own category, but note that the pigmented phytonutrients mentioned above, such as carotenoids, anthocyanins, and chlorophyll, are part of the reason to categorize fruits into their own food group.

In addition to their pigments, fruits are very similar to vegetables, and research typically lumps them together, as the recommendations from worldwide health organizations are to increase both fruit and vegetable consumption to mitigate unnecessary disease and early mortality. The World Health Organization estimates that nearly four million deaths could be attributed to suboptimal fruit and vegetable consumption worldwide in 2017, and recommends including 400 grams of vegetables and fruits per day to improve health and decrease disease risk.[23]

To individuate some highlights, here are some ways to categorize fruits:

- *Berries* include blueberries, blackberries, raspberries, strawberries, cranberries, and currants and are small, juicy, antioxidant-rich fruits grown on bushes and vines. Berries are great dietary sources of bioactive compounds, phenolic compounds such as phenolic acids, flavonoids-flavonols, anthocyanins, tannins, and ascorbic acid that may act as strong anti-oxidants and could help in the prevention of inflammatory disorders and cardiovascular diseases, and lower the risk of various cancers.

- *Citrus fruits* include grapefruits, lemons, limes, kumquats, oranges, and tangerines, and are characterized by a thick rind, most of which is a bitter white pith known as *albedo,* covered by a thin, colored skin known as the *zest.* Citrus fruits offer dietary fiber and vitamin C, and are a source of B vitamins (thiamin, pyridoxine, niacin, riboflavin, pantothenic acid, and folate), and phytochemicals, such as carotenoids, flavonoids, and limonoids.

- *Stone fruits*, also known as *drupes,* include apricots, cherries, peaches, nectarines, and plums, and are characterized by thin skin, soft flesh, and a single woody stone or pit. These fruits contain anthocyanins and other phenolic compounds associated with antioxidant, anti-inflammatory, and antimicrobial activities.

- *Tropical or exotic fruits* are native to regions around the world with hot, tropical, and subtropical terrain, though they are available for consumption worldwide. The most commonly consumed tropical fruits are bananas, dates, kiwi, passion fruit, mango, papaya, pineapple, and jackfruit, and those becoming more widely familiar include rambutan, lychee, cherimoya, mangosteen, durian, custard apple, dragonfruit, longan, guava, and star fruit.

- *Pomes* or *tree fruits*, such as apples, pears, and quince, contain a central core with many small seeds and thin skin with firm flesh.

- *Melons* are members of the gourd family and include cantaloupe, honeydew, casaba melon, crenshaw melon, Santa Claus melon, watermelon, red seedless watermelon, and gold watermelon. They are approximately 90 percent water but still high in fiber, vitamin C, and carotenoids.

Three servings of fruits per day include 1 medium piece or 1 cup.

Nuts and Seeds

Nuts and seeds are exceptionally nutrient-dense nuggets that support weight loss and weight-loss maintenance.[24,25,26,27,28,29] Nuts and seeds are concentrated in unique nutrients and bioactive compounds, including fiber; amino acids such as L-arginine; monounsaturated and polyunsaturated fats (and, bonus, they are low in saturated fats); vitamins E, K, folate, and thiamine; essential minerals, including calcium, copper, iron, magnesium, phosphorus, potassium, selenium, and zinc; and phytonutrients such as phytosterols, beta-sitosterol, lignans, and ellagic acid.[30] Consuming nuts and seeds is also associated with improved satiety, insulin sensitivity, cholesterol profiles, and cognitive function; and a reduced risk of cardiovascular disease and mortality.[31,32,33,34,35,36]

Aim to consume between 1 to 2 ounces (30 to 40 grams) of nuts and seeds per day. The best way to do so is by using them as a base for a dressing or sauce to enjoy over vegetables. This makes it easier to eat more veggies, encourages absorption of the fat-soluble nutrients, and helps mitigate hand-to-mouth noshing that is common with this food group. For the recipes in this book, feel free to swap out other nuts or seeds in the dressings and sauces for variety.

This category includes tree nuts, which encompass almonds, Brazil nuts, cashews, hazelnuts, macadamias, pecans, pistachios, and walnuts; legume seeds, such as peanuts; and other seeds, such as chia, flax, hemp, poppy, pumpkin, sesame, and sunflower.

Legumes

Legumes include all the vast varieties of beans, lentils, peas, hummus (which should be a food group of its own because it is so versatile, nutritious, and delicious), and soyfoods such as tofu and tempeh. This category is highlighted because these foods are a rich source of essential amino acids and fibers, including resistant starch, soluble, and insoluble. They are high in the minerals iron, calcium, zinc, magnesium, phosphorus, potassium, and manganese, as well as B vitamins (especially folate), and phytonutrients, including isoflavones, flavonoids, lignans, lutein, and zeaxanthin.

Consuming legumes has been positively associated with optimized weight management; decreased risk for cardiovascular disease by lowering blood lipids and improving vascular function and insulin sensitivity; decreased risk of type 2 diabetes via better glycemic control; and decreased risk of certain cancers via anti-inflammatory and antioxidant effects.[37,38,39,40]

Opt for approximately 1 to 1½ cups of legumes per day. Try them in the Sweet Potato Dal (page 57), Smoky Split Pea Stew (page 69), Zuppa Toscana (page 64), Saag Paneer (page 98), and Fresh Butter Bean Smash Lettuce Wraps (page 117) as delicious options.

Mushrooms

Mushrooms, part of the fungi family, have been consumed as food and medicine for millennia, and there are myriad reasons to prioritize them in a healthy diet. Despite being very low in calories, they are uniquely rich in multiple bioactive compounds such as several phytochemicals including alkaloids, carotenoids, flavonoids, and phenolic acids; different fibers, such as beta-glucans, hemicelluloses, and pectins; minerals, especially selenium, copper, potassium, phosphorus, calcium, iron, and zinc; and certain vitamins, including riboflavin, niacin, and folate. When wild or irradiated with UV light, they can be considered the only source for vitamin D that is not based on consuming animal products or exposure to sunlight. They are also high in the antioxidant glutathione and the cytoprotective and disease-fighting amino acid, ergothioneine.[41,42,43,44]

The medicinal properties of mushrooms include being antioxidant, anti-inflammatory, antidiabetic, antiallergic, immunomodulating, cardioprotective, cholesterol-lowering, antiviral, antibacterial, antiparasitic, antifungal, detoxifying, and protective against cancer.[45,46]

Choose amongst the many edible species, including shiitake, oyster, maitake, king oyster, white button, cremini, portobello, enoki, porcini, and chanterelle. Enjoy at least three different varieties each week. In the recipe chapters ahead, you can find many magical mushroom options highlighted in Mighty Mushroom Miso Soup (page 70), Creamy Mushroom Soup (page 72), Autumnal Stuffed Mushrooms (page 88), Immunity Bowl (page 134), and Polenta with Red Wine Glazed Mushrooms (page 141).

Overall, the 6 Daily 3's are the most health-promoting foods, offering unique nutrient profiles, and should form the foundation of your diet. Once you have accounted for these foods, add more of them–as well as whole grains–as needed for culinary diversity and to maintain adequate calories and your comfortable weight.

Sustainability

Now that you have set your boundaries and see the broader picture of what the long-term diet looks like, continue using any of the tools that worked during weight loss–maintain a food journal, refer to the emotion to-do lists, and keep sticky notes or other reminders around. Here are some additional tools you can utilize throughout your journey to stay focused and to maintain mindfulness.

Gratitude List

What are you grateful for? Right now, in this moment, what do you appreciate? Take a moment and start a list of all the things you are grateful for. Not the list that begins once you achieve your goal weight. Instead, it is the gratitude you feel now. This can include little things (cozy slippers, a mug of tea, a hot bath) as well as big things (family, health and the health of those you love, relationships with friends). As long as they are significant to you, include them in your list. Nothing is too trivial.

My clients have told me about their gratitude lists, which often include things like *I can sit down on the floor to play with my grandchild; I can walk up the stairs without getting out of breath; I enjoy my food so much more, my confidence has increased; food does not intimidate me anymore*; and so many others.

Keep this as an ongoing, exhaustive list. (I keep mine in my notes on my phone so I can add to it whenever I think of something.) It may seem inconsequential, but having this in writing is certainly empowering.

Days of Deliciousness

The popular concept of allowing for a "cheat day" has such an interestingly negative connotation. Cheating, by definition, implies you are violating rules or acting unfaithfully. With respect to a diet, cheating alludes to feeling like you are in a state of restriction and suffering, craving an opportunity to deviate from your plan.

What if we flip this thinking on its head completely? What if our way of eating consists of foods we love to eat every day, so no cheat day is required? Once your palate adjusts to eating whole foods, enjoying your meals should come naturally, and because of the results you achieve on your weight-loss and health outcomes, eating this way becomes a beloved and conscientiously chosen priority.

Once in a while, there can be room to schedule times for an indulgence, a *day of deliciousness* (or a day for *extra* deliciousness). Occasions such as a friend coming to visit, you or your loved one celebrating a milestone, or a special holiday that is sentimental to you may call for a specific indulgent food or meal. If you choose these with purpose and planning rather than just letting them happen or become a regular part of your routine, they will be exactly as they were intended–a special treat. What you do over the majority of your days, weeks, and months are what will have the direct and overt impact on your weight and health. An occasional day of deliciousness will not derail you.

Choose Again

Long-term behavioral changes and weight management require ongoing, persistent attention.[47] But with these strategies outlined in this chapter and a continued focus on your why, you can successfully maintain this achievement throughout your life.

Everything happens in *this* moment. You have an opportunity to choose each time. Based on whether this decision is on-plan, whether it serves you in this moment, and what the implications will be; choose to stay on-plan. Choose to pursue your why.

Tomorrow, next week, and next month will arrive no matter what. Where do you want to be at those points in time? Do you want to tell yourself that you will start next Monday, next week, or next month? Or do you want to be in the throes of it, making progress, enjoying the fruits of your focus? You get to decide. You get to choose you now. It's the perfect time, and you have everything you need. Nothing and nobody can stop you.

Choose you now.

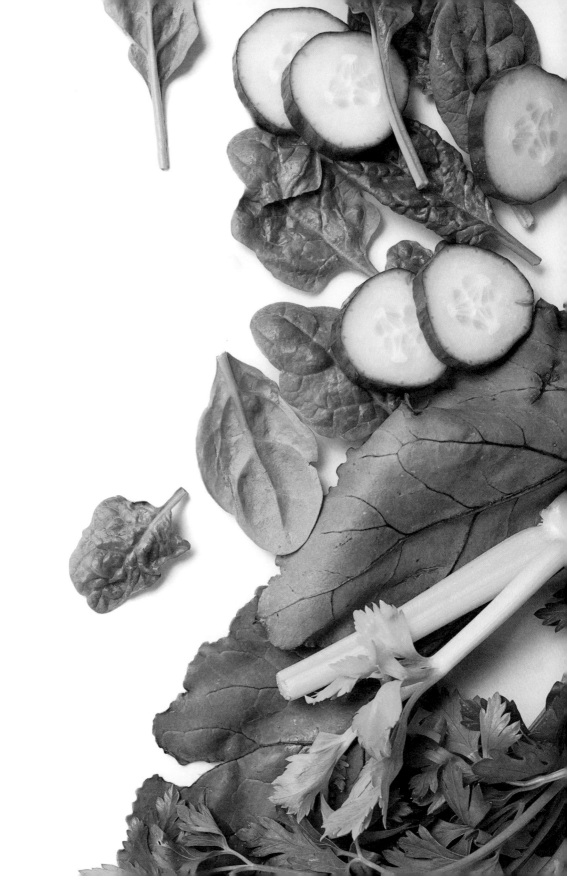

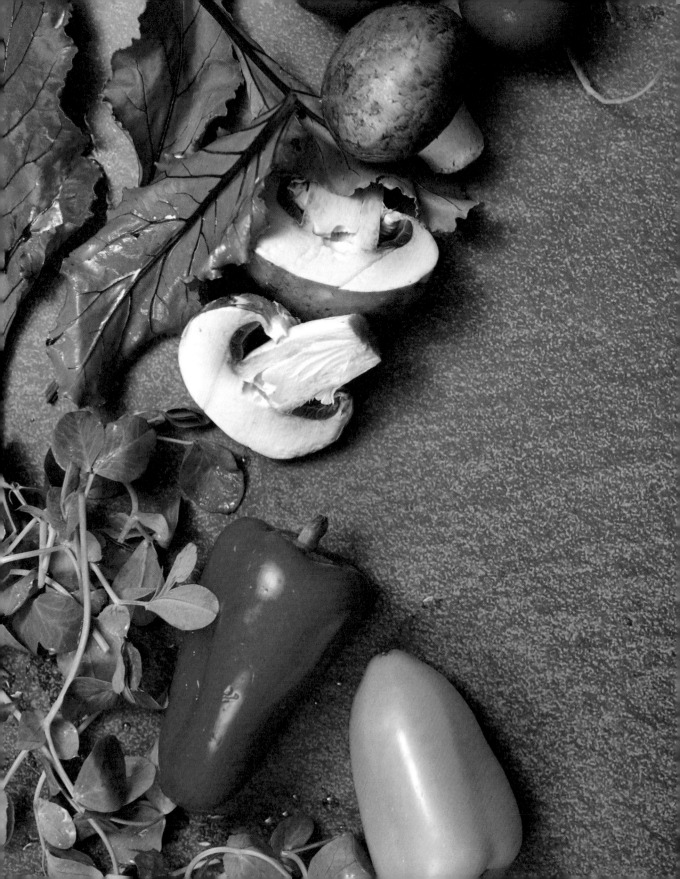

CHAPTER 6
POTS

Thai Green Curry

One of my favorite dishes from Thailand is green curry; the flavors and textures vary depending on where you find it, but it's always delicious. In this version, the traditional coconut milk is replaced with plant milk and a bit of coconut extract, which saves a bunch of saturated fat grams but retains the dish's classic essence.

½ cup raw cashews
4 tbsp green curry paste (look for a vegan, low-sodium option)
½ tsp coconut extract (see note)
1 cup plant milk
1 shallot, thinly sliced
1 jalapeño, chopped
1 red bell pepper, thinly sliced
1 small sweet potato, peeled and sliced
1 small Japanese eggplant, sliced
1 carrot, cut into rounds
2 cups low-sodium vegetable broth
1 medium head bok choy, chopped
1 cup sliced mushrooms (cremini, oyster, maitake, or button)
1 cup broccoli florets, chopped small
Juice of ½ lime
Lime wedges, to garnish
½ cup fresh Thai basil (or basil or cilantro), to garnish

1. In a blender, combine the cashews, curry paste, coconut extract, and plant milk. Blend until smooth, and set aside.

2. Heat a large saucepan or Dutch oven over medium-high heat. When hot, sauté the shallot with as little water as possible, just enough to avoid burning, for 3 minutes or until translucent.

3. Add the jalapeño and bell pepper, and sauté with additional water as needed for 2 minutes or until the vegetables are soft. Add the sweet potato, eggplant, carrot, and broth; and bring to a boil. When boiling, lower the heat, and simmer for 10 minutes or until the vegetables soften.

4. Add the bok choy, mushrooms, broccoli, and cashew cream. Return to a boil, and then reduce the heat and simmer for 10 minutes more until the vegetables are cooked but still a vibrant green. Stir in the lime juice. Garnish with lime wedges and Thai basil, and serve hot.

> NOTE Coconut extract is available online, and a small bottle will last a long time.

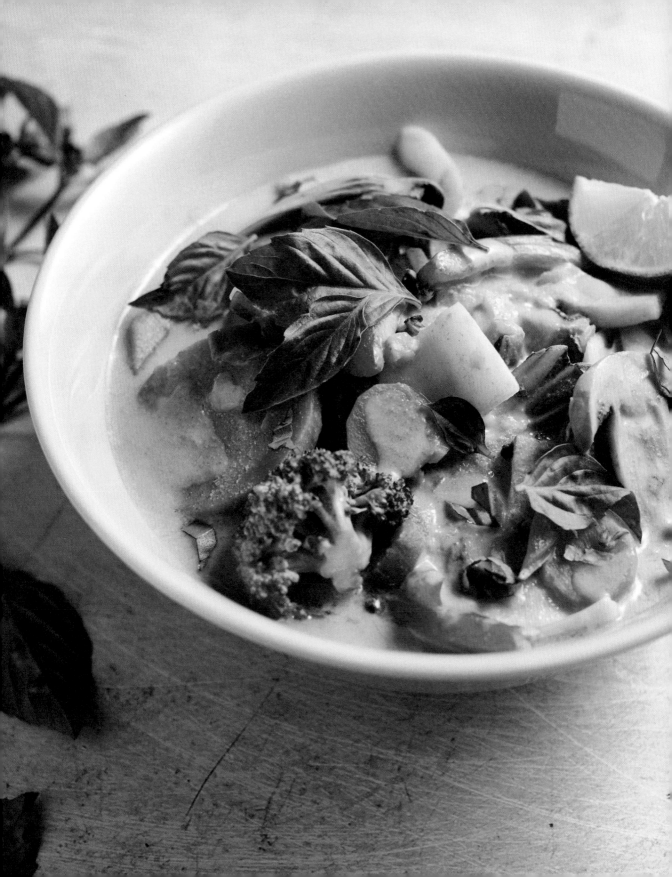

Prep Time: 10 minutes

Cook Time: 1 hour 10 minutes

Serves: 4–8

Comfort Chili con Quinoa

Quinoa and beans add a meaty consistency to this hearty chili. Keep a batch on hand in the refrigerator or freezer for a wholesome meal anytime. For extra pizazz, top with a spicy cheese sauce, such as Sweet Potato Cheesy Sauce (page 163) or Nacho Squash Sauce (page 165). It also makes a great topping over brown or black rice, quinoa, a baked potato, or a bed of greens.

1 cup quinoa, rinsed

1½ cups water

1 white or yellow onion, diced

1 jalapeño or serrano, diced with seeds (remove seeds or omit pepper for less heat)

1 green bell pepper, diced

4 cloves garlic, minced

3 tbsp chili powder (reduce for less heat)

1 tbsp ground cumin

1 tbsp smoked paprika

1 tsp chipotle powder

¼–½ tsp cayenne

1 (15oz; 425g) can kidney beans, mostly drained

1 (15oz; 425g) can black beans, mostly drained

2 cups low-sodium vegetable broth

1 cup crushed tomatoes

4 tbsp tomato paste

2–3 tbsp reduced-sodium tamari

Chopped fresh parsley or cilantro, to garnish

1. To a small saucepan, add the quinoa, and toast over medium heat until the quinoa is dry from the rinse and begins to toast. Add the water, and bring to a boil. Reduce the heat, cover, and simmer on low for 10 to 15 minutes until all the water is absorbed. When the water is absorbed, remove from the heat, keep covered, and allow the quinoa to steam for 5 minutes. Fluff with a fork and set aside.

2. Heat a large saucepan or Dutch oven over medium-high heat. When hot, sauté the onion with as little water as possible, just enough to avoid burning, for 3 minutes or until translucent.

3. Add the jalapeño and bell pepper, and cook for 2 to 3 minutes until the vegetables soften, adding water as needed, and stirring occasionally. Add the garlic, chili powder, cumin, paprika, chipotle powder, and cayenne. Sauté for 60 to 90 seconds, being careful to brown but not burn.

4. Add the kidney beans, black beans, broth, tomatoes, and tomato paste; and stir to combine. Bring to a boil. Reduce the heat, cover, and simmer on low for 40 to 50 minutes, stirring occasionally, until the sauce has thickened.

5. Add the quinoa and tamari, stir, and adjust seasonings as desired. Serve hot, garnished with parsley or cilantro.

Sweet Potato Dal

Prep Time: 10 minutes
Cook Time: 45–55 minutes
Serves: 2–4

Red lentils deliver silky smooth decadence with extraordinary nutrition—fiber, folate, iron, zinc, phosphorus, magnesium, potassium . . . shall I go on? Together with sweet potato, they make a lovely, satisfying stew. For a balanced meal, serve this dal with a side salad of cucumber, red onion, tomato, and cilantro, dressed with a splash of lemon juice.

1 cup finely chopped yellow or red onion

1 jalapeño (or serrano or bird's-eye chile), deseeded and finely chopped

1 medium sweet potato, peeled and diced small

3 cloves garlic, minced

½ tbsp minced fresh ginger

1 cup red lentils, rinsed

2 tsp ground cumin

2 tsp ground coriander

2 tsp garam masala

1 tsp ground turmeric

1 (15oz; 425g) can crushed tomatoes

4 cups low-sodium vegetable broth

¼ cup (packed) fresh cilantro, chopped

2 tsp reduced-sodium tamari (optional)

1. Heat a medium saucepan over medium-high heat. When hot, sauté the onion with as little water as possible, just enough to avoid burning, for 3 minutes or until translucent.

2. Add the jalapeño and a few tablespoons of water (if needed to avoid burning), and sauté for 1 minute. Add the sweet potatoes and additional water as necessary, and cook for 5 minutes.

3. Add the garlic and ginger, and cook for 30 seconds, stirring frequently. Add the lentils, cumin, coriander, garam masala, and turmeric; and stir to combine. Stir in the tomatoes and broth, and bring to a boil. When boiling, reduce the heat, and simmer on low for 25 to 35 minutes until the potatoes and lentils are soft. Stir in the cilantro and tamari, if using. Serve hot.

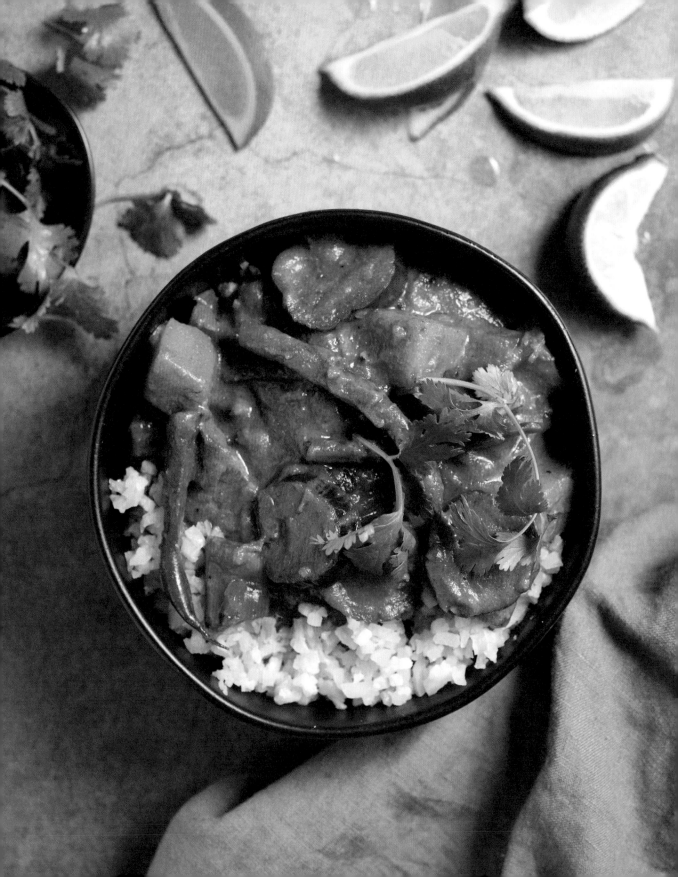

Peanut Butter Vegetable Curry

Prep Time: 15 minutes
Cook Time: 30–40 minutes
Serves: 2–4

If there is one way to make veggies more enticing, it is to add peanut butter. This hearty array of vegetables mixed with warm, spicy curry seasonings and the creamy goodness of peanut butter makes for a simple, comforting treat. (P.S. Nobody would think of this as a "weight-loss" food, so have it at the ready when you are hosting guests and trying to impress.)

1 cup chopped yellow onion

1 tbsp finely minced jalapeño

2 cloves garlic, minced

1 tsp minced fresh ginger

2 tsp curry powder

1 tsp ground cumin

1 tsp smoked paprika

½ tsp cayenne

1 medium Japanese eggplant, sliced

1 cup fresh green beans, trimmed and halved

1 small red bell pepper, chopped

1 cup chopped kabocha or butternut squash

1 (14.5oz; 411g) can no-salt-added, fire-roasted diced tomatoes

2 cups low-sodium vegetable broth

¼ cup tomato paste

¼ cup peanut butter

2 tbsp reduced-sodium tamari

1 tbsp freshly squeezed lime juice

1 tsp liquid smoke

½ cup chopped fresh cilantro, plus more to garnish

Cooked brown rice or cauliflower rice (optional), to serve

Harissa powder (optional), to garnish

1. Heat a large saucepan or Dutch oven over medium-high heat. When hot, sauté the onion with as little water as possible, just enough to avoid burning, for 3 minutes or until translucent. Add the jalapeño, garlic, ginger, curry powder, cumin, paprika, and cayenne, along with 1 to 2 tablespoons water; and cook for 1 minute more, stirring frequently.

2. Add the eggplant, green beans, bell pepper, kabocha, tomatoes, broth, tomato paste, and peanut butter; and bring to a boil over medium-high heat. When boiling, reduce the heat to low, and simmer for 20 to 30 minutes until the vegetables are tender. Add the tamari, lime juice, and liquid smoke. Taste and adjust the seasonings as needed. Remove from the heat, and stir in the cilantro.

3. Serve warm over brown rice or cauliflower rice, if using, and garnish with harissa powder and additional cilantro, if desired.

Jambalaya Oats

Jambalaya is traditionally a Creole dish made with rice, vegetables, spices, and smoked meat. Here, oat groats replace rice for an even more nutritious, healthful option but with a very similar texture, and a dash of liquid smoke is used instead of meat. Oat groats are the whole oat with just the hulls removed, so they are a fantastic source of fiber, vitamins, and minerals.

1 cup chopped
  yellow onion
3 cloves garlic, minced
1 red bell pepper,
  chopped
2 celery stalks, chopped
1 cup oat groats, rinsed
1 (14.5oz; 411g) can
  no-salt-added,
  fire-roasted diced
  tomatoes
¼ cup tomato paste
1 (15oz; 425g) can red
  kidney beans, drained
  and rinsed
2 tbsp Cajun Spice
  Blend (see note) or
  salt-free Cajun
  seasoning
1 bay leaf
2½ cups low-sodium
  vegetable broth
1 tbsp anchovy-free
  Worcestershire sauce
1 tsp liquid smoke
Hot sauce (optional),
  to taste
Freshly ground black
  pepper, to taste
½ cup chopped fresh
  parsley, to garnish

1. Heat a large saucepan or Dutch oven over medium-high heat. When hot, sauté the onion with as little water as possible, just enough to avoid burning, until translucent and beginning to caramelize.

2. Add the garlic, and cook for 30 to 45 seconds until golden brown. Add the bell pepper and celery, and cook until the vegetables soften, adding 1 tablespoon of water at a time to avoid burning. Add the oat groats, tomatoes, tomato paste, kidney beans, Cajun Spice Blend, bay leaf, and broth; and bring to a boil. When boiling, cover, reduce the heat to low, and simmer for 45 minutes, stirring occasionally, or until all the liquid is absorbed and the stew thickens.

3. Add the Worcestershire and liquid smoke, and stir to combine. Remove the bay leaf, and add hot sauce and pepper, if desired. Garnish with parsley, and serve immediately.

NOTE To make **Cajun Spice Blend,** in a small bowl, mix together the following: 2½ tsp dried thyme, 2 tsp garlic powder, 2 tsp smoked paprika, 1 tsp onion powder, 1 tsp dried oregano, 1 tsp red pepper flakes or cayenne, ½ tsp freshly ground black pepper. Transfer to an airtight jar for storage.

Curried Parsnip Purée

Prep Time: 20 minutes
Cook Time: 60 minutes
Serves: 2-4

Roasting parsnips caramelizes them, bringing out their most amazing nutty, sweet, buttery flavors. These superb starchy root veggies shine as the main attraction in this curry purée.

24oz (680g) parsnips, peeled and chopped into 1-in (2.5cm) pieces (see note)
1 small yellow onion, chopped
2 cloves garlic, minced
1 tsp minced fresh ginger
2 tsp curry powder
1 tsp ground cumin
½ tsp ground coriander
¼–½ tsp red pepper flakes
1 cup cauliflower rice
2 cups low-sodium vegetable broth
½ tbsp miso paste
½ cup plant milk
Arugula leaves, to garnish

1. Preheat the oven to 400°F (200°C). Line a baking sheet with parchment paper or a silicone baking mat. Spread the parsnips on the prepared baking sheet, and bake for 40 minutes until golden brown, flipping them after 20 minutes. Set aside.

2. Heat a large saucepan or Dutch oven over medium-high heat. When hot, sauté the onion with as little water as possible, just enough to avoid burning, for 3 minutes or until translucent. Add the garlic and ginger, and sauté for 30 seconds, adding a splash of water as needed to avoid burning. Add the curry powder, cumin, coriander, and red pepper flakes; and toast for 1 minute, adding a splash of water if needed.

3. Add the roasted parsnips, cauliflower rice, and broth. Bring to a boil. When boiling, reduce the heat to low, and simmer for 15 minutes or until the parsnips are softened. Remove from the heat, and stir in the miso paste and milk. Transfer to a blender or use an immersion blender in the pot, and purée to your desired texture—slightly chunky or velvety smooth. Serve hot, garnished with fresh arugula.

NOTE Peel some parsnip curls with a vegetable peeler before chopping the parsnips. Add the curls to the baking sheet in the last 10 minutes of baking for a crispy, curly garnish to serve.

Creamy Potato Corn Chowder

Creamy potatoes combined with sweet yellow corn and the freshness of dill make for a lovely, satiating pot of deliciousness. Peel the potatoes, if you prefer, and add some "nooch" (nutritional yeast) for a boost of umami.

1 yellow onion, diced
3 celery stalks, chopped
3 carrots, chopped
1 green bell pepper, chopped
4 cloves garlic, minced
4 cups low-sodium vegetable broth, divided
4 medium Yukon Gold potatoes, cubed
2 cups frozen corn
1 bay leaf
1 tsp freshly ground black pepper
4 tbsp chopped fresh dill, divided
3 tbsp reduced-sodium tamari
2 cups plant milk
1 tbsp freshly squeezed lemon juice
1 tbsp nutritional yeast (optional)

1. Heat a large saucepan or Dutch oven over medium-high heat. When hot, sauté the onion with as little water as possible, just enough to avoid burning, for 3 minutes or until translucent.

2. Add the celery, carrots, bell pepper, garlic, and 1 cup broth. Cook for 5 minutes or until the vegetables begin to soften. Stir in the remaining 3 cups broth, potatoes, corn, bay leaf, pepper, and 2 tablespoons dill. Bring to a boil. When boiling, reduce the heat to medium-low, cover, and simmer for 15 to 20 minutes until the vegetables are soft.

3. Stir in the tamari and plant milk, return to a boil, and cook for 5 to 10 minutes. Turn off the heat, and remove the bay leaf. With an immersion blender, blend the soup until mostly puréed but slightly chunky (or to your preferred texture).

4. Return the pot to medium-high heat, and cook for 5 to 10 minutes until thickened. Add the remaining 2 tablespoons dill, lemon juice, and nutritional yeast, if using; and stir to combine. Serve hot.

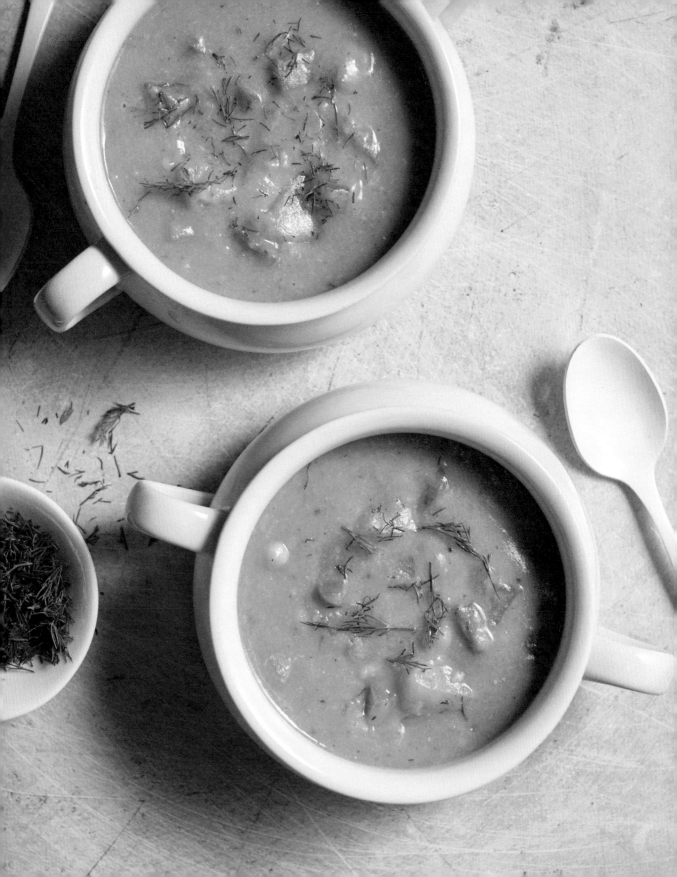

Prep Time: 20 minutes
Cook Time: 40 minutes
Serves: 3–4

Zuppa Toscana
(Italian White Bean and Tomato Soup)

A soup from Tuscany, traditionally made with a combination of vegetables, potatoes, white beans, and kale. This dish is simple, satisfying, and classic.

1 yellow onion, chopped

4 cloves garlic, minced

2 roasted red peppers (jarred in water), chopped

3 small russet potatoes, peeled and chopped

1 (15oz; 425g) can cannellini beans, drained and rinsed

1 (28oz; 794g) can crushed tomatoes

2 tbsp tomato paste

3 cups low-sodium vegetable broth

½ cup nutritional yeast

½ cup plant milk

1 tbsp reduced-sodium tamari

2 bay leaves

1 tsp Italian seasoning

½ tsp red pepper flakes

½ tsp freshly ground black pepper

4 cups chopped lacinato (Tuscan) kale

½ cup packed chopped fresh basil, divided, plus more to garnish

1. Heat a large saucepan or Dutch oven over medium-high heat. When hot, sauté the onion with as little water as possible, just enough to avoid burning, for 3 minutes or until translucent. Add the garlic, and sauté for 30 to 60 seconds or until golden, being careful not to scorch.

2. Stir in the roasted red peppers, potatoes, beans, tomatoes, tomato paste, broth, nutritional yeast, plant milk, tamari, bay leaves, Italian seasoning, red pepper flakes, pepper, kale, and half of the basil. Bring to a boil over medium-high heat. Reduce the heat, cover, and simmer for 30 minutes or until the potatoes are fork-tender, stirring occasionally.

3. Turn off the heat, remove the bay leaves, and add the remaining basil. Stir to combine, and serve hot with additional basil chiffonade as a garnish, if desired.

Hearty Butternut and Millet Stew with Fresh Dill

Prep Time: 10 minutes
Cook Time: 40–50 minutes
Serves: 3–4

Millet is a gluten-free seed grass that has been enjoyed by humans for thousands of years. This underappreciated staple has a mild flavor and lovely chewy texture that makes this stew seem like a savory porridge.

1 sweet yellow onion, chopped
2 tsp ground turmeric
1 tsp ground cumin
1 tsp red pepper flakes
4 carrots, sliced into ¾-in (2cm) pieces
3 celery stalks, sliced into ¾-in (2cm) pieces
2 cups chopped butternut squash
1 (15oz; 425g) can chickpeas, drained and rinsed
3 medium russet potatoes, chopped
1 cup millet
4 cups low-sodium vegetable broth
4 cups water
½ cup chopped fresh dill, divided
1 tbsp freshly squeezed lemon juice
1 tsp reduced-sodium tamari
¼ tsp freshly ground black pepper
Aleppo powder or paprika (optional), to garnish

1. Heat a large saucepan or Dutch oven over medium-high heat. When hot, sauté the onion with as little water as possible, just enough to avoid burning, for 3 minutes or until translucent. Add the turmeric, cumin, and red pepper flakes; and cook for 1 minute. Add the carrots, celery, squash, chickpeas, potatoes, millet, broth, water, and half of the dill.

2. Bring to a boil over high heat. When boiling, reduce the heat to low, and simmer, partially covered, for 30 to 40 minutes until the vegetables are tender.

3. Turn off the heat. Stir in the lemon juice, tamari, and pepper along with the remaining dill. Serve hot, with a sprinkle of Aleppo powder or paprika to garnish, if using, or allow to cool and refrigerate in an airtight container for up to 6 days.

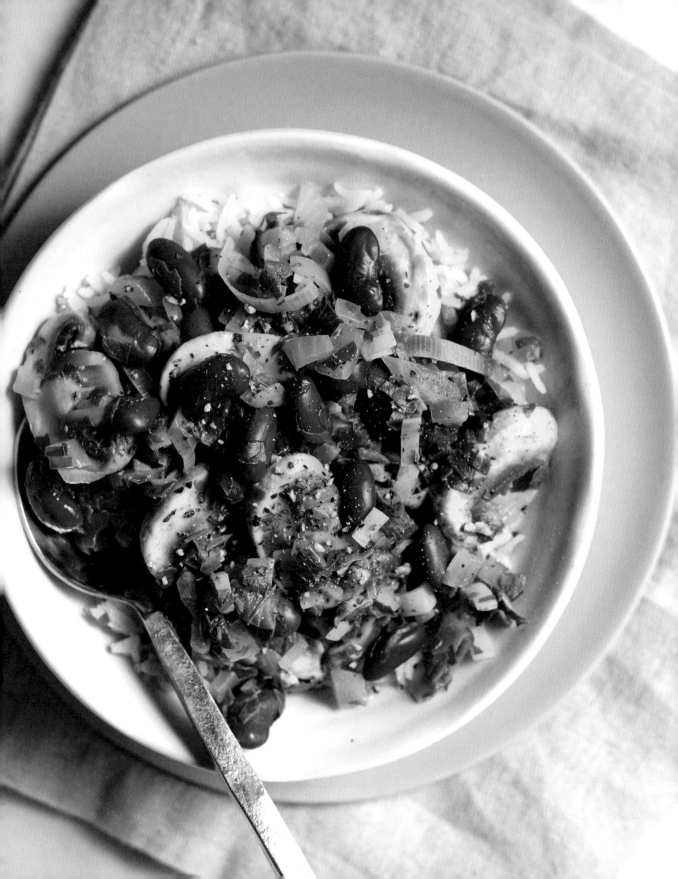

Khoresh-e Ghormeh Sabzi
(Persian Fresh Herb Stew)

Prep Time: 15 minutes
Cook Time: 40 minutes
Serves: 2

This recipe was inspired by one of my best friends in the world, who makes a similar Persian stew, brimming with flavor, for her family holiday parties. Traditionally, *ghormeh sabzi* features meat and sour, dried Persian limes (which work deliciously in this recipe if you can find them), but adding the peel of a lime while simmering and finishing with lime juice replicates the tart and pungent flavor of the original dish.

1 cup chopped fresh spinach
1 cup chopped fresh cilantro
1 cup chopped flat-leaf parsley
1 leek, cleaned well and roughly chopped
2 limes
1 large yellow onion, sliced
2 cups sliced cremini mushrooms
1 tbsp dried fenugreek
½ tsp freshly ground black pepper
½ tsp ground turmeric
½ tsp ground cinnamon
2 cups low-sodium vegetable broth
1 (15oz; 425g) can kidney beans, drained and rinsed

1. In a food processor, pulse the spinach, cilantro, parsley, and leeks to a fine chop, and set aside.

2. Using a vegetable peeler, remove large strips of zest from 1 lime, stripping away about half of the green surface area. Halve the lime, and squeeze the juice into a small bowl. Juice the remaining lime into the same bowl. (You should have about 4–6 tablespoons lime juice.) Set aside the strips of zest and the juice.

3. Heat a large saucepan or Dutch oven over medium-high heat. When hot, sauté the onion with as little water as possible, just enough to avoid burning, for 3 minutes or until translucent. Add the mushrooms, cover, and cook for 3 to 4 minutes until their liquid is released. Add the fenugreek, pepper, turmeric, and cinnamon, and sauté for 2 minutes more.

4. Transfer the chopped greens to the pot, and cook, stirring frequently, for about 5 minutes. Add the broth, beans, lime zest, and 2 to 3 tablespoons lime juice. Reduce the heat to low, and simmer for 20 minutes. Stir in the remaining lime juice, remove the strips of zest, and serve hot.

> NOTE Traditionally, this dish is served over white basmati rice, like other Persian stews, but this version is delicious over a baked potato or whole grains.

Prep Time: 10 minutes
Cook Time: 30 minutes
Serves: 4

Tempeh and Potato Stew

Like a hug in a bowl! A hearty, simple stew featuring potatoes and tempeh—an Indonesian fermented soy food—surrounded by other kitchen staples, including frozen pearl onions, peas, and tomato paste. Red wine and spices add richness and flavor.

1 (8oz; 227g) pkg tempeh, cubed
2 cups cubed potatoes
1 cup frozen petite pearl onions
1 cup diced carrots
1 cup diced celery
2 tbsp tomato paste
2 tbsp reduced-sodium tamari
2 tbsp anchovy-free Worcestershire sauce
1 tsp garlic powder
1 tsp onion powder
1 tsp dried basil
1 tsp dried oregano
1 bay leaf
1 tsp freshly ground black pepper
3 cups low-sodium vegetable broth
1 cup frozen peas
½ cup red wine
2 tbsp chickpea flour or arrowroot powder
2 tbsp water
¼ cup chopped fresh flat-leaf parsley

1. To a large saucepan or Dutch oven, add the tempeh, potatoes, onions, carrots, celery, tomato paste, tamari, Worcestershire, garlic powder, onion powder, basil, oregano, bay leaf, pepper, and broth. Bring to a boil over medium-high heat. When boiling, reduce the heat to medium-low, cover, and simmer for 20 minutes or until the vegetables are tender.

2. Add the peas and red wine, stir to combine, and simmer for 2 minutes more. In a small bowl, whisk together the chickpea flour and water to make a slurry. Add the slurry to the pot, stir, and simmer for 5 minutes or until the stew is thickened.

3. Remove from the heat, remove the bay leaf, and stir in the parsley. Serve immediately, or allow to cool and store in an airtight container for up to 5 days in the refrigerator.

Smoky Split Pea Stew

Prep Time: 20 minutes
Cook Time: 1 hour 10 minutes
Serves: 6–8

Classic comfort food with extraordinary nutritional gravitas! With optimal levels of fiber, folate, iron, potassium, phosphorus, magnesium, and zinc, split peas are an ideal ingredient as the main attraction, backed up by creamy potatoes and a hit of liquid smoke for a super-satiating staple meal.

1 yellow onion, chopped
2 cloves garlic, minced
3 carrots, diced
3 stalks celery, chopped
1 medium celery root (celeriac), chopped
2 cups dried split peas, rinsed
3 medium Yukon Gold potatoes, coarsely chopped
7 cups water
1 bay leaf
1 tsp celery seed
1 tsp dried parsley
1 tsp dried thyme
1 tsp dried rosemary
½ tsp freshly ground black pepper
2 tbsp reduced-sodium tamari
1 tbsp freshly squeezed lemon juice
1½ tsp liquid smoke or smoked paprika, to taste

1. Heat a large saucepan or Dutch oven over medium-high heat. When hot, sauté the onion with as little water as possible, just enough to avoid burning, for 3 minutes or until translucent. Add the garlic, carrots, celery, and celery root, and cook for 2 minutes more.

2. Add the peas, potatoes, and water to the pot. Stir in the bay leaf, celery seed, parsley, thyme, rosemary, and pepper. Bring to a boil over high heat. When boiling, reduce the heat to medium-low and simmer, partially covered, for 50 to 60 minutes until the peas are soft. Stir in the tamari, lemon juice, and liquid smoke.

3. Once the peas are tender, taste and adjust the seasonings as desired. Cook for 3 to 5 minutes, uncovered, to thicken. (Or add water to thin.) Remove the bay leaf and serve immediately, or allow to cool and refrigerate in an airtight container for up to 6 days.

Mighty Mushroom Miso Soup

Prep Time: 10 minutes
Cook Time: 10–15 minutes
Serves: 2–4

As a young girl, I toured in Japan with a theatre company and had the opportunity to stay with host families in Tokyo and Kyoto. It was my first exposure to traditional Japanese diets, and I was impressed and excited by the idea of enjoying miso soup and rice three times a day. Rich in probiotics, miso soup is considered good for digestion. This recipe bulks up a simple traditional soup with extra mushrooms, zucchini noodles, and bok choy to make a heartier, more satisfying meal.

3 tbsp wakame
16oz (450g) shiitake mushrooms, sliced
1 tsp reduced-sodium tamari
6 cups low-sodium vegetable broth
3 scallions, sliced
2 cups zucchini noodles
4 cups thinly sliced baby bok choy
2 tbsp miso paste
1 tsp sesame seeds (optional), to garnish
Togarashi (optional), to garnish

1. In a medium bowl, soak the wakame in hot water for 5 minutes. Drain, squeeze to remove excess water, and set aside.

2. Place a large saucepan over medium-high heat. Add the mushrooms and 2 to 3 tablespoons water, cover, and cook for 3 to 5 minutes until the mushrooms release liquid and it begins to bubble. Once bubbling, remove the cover, add the tamari, and cook for 3 to 5 minutes, stirring frequently, until the mushrooms start to brown. Add a little water, if necessary, to prevent burning.

3. Add the broth, scallions, zucchini noodles, and bok choy; and bring to a boil. Once boiling, stir in the soaked and drained wakame, and turn off the heat.

4. In a small bowl, combine the miso paste with ½ cup of hot broth from the pot, and stir to dissolve. Add the miso mixture to the pot, stir to combine, and serve hot. Garnish with sesame seeds and togarashi, if desired.

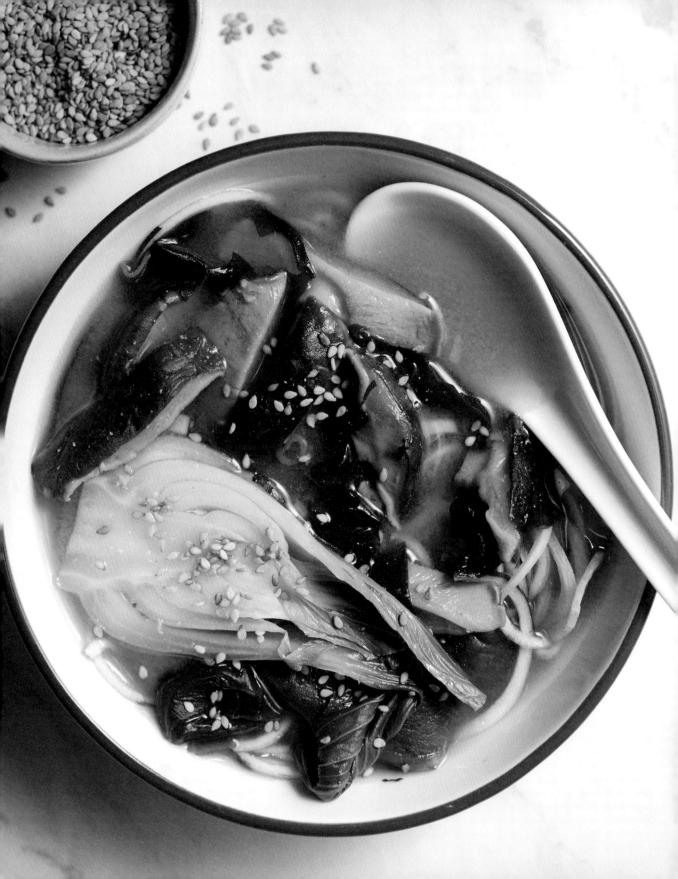

Prep Time: 20 minutes
Cook Time: 25–35 minutes
Serves: 2–4

Creamy Mushroom Soup

Cream of mushroom soup reinvented! Loaded with hearty mushrooms and made with a rich hemp seed cream sauce, this flavorful soul-soothing soup is a staple in my home.

½ cup hemp seeds
4 tbsp nutritional yeast
1 tbsp freshly squeezed lemon juice
1 tbsp apple cider vinegar
1 tbsp anchovy-free Worcestershire sauce
1 tbsp reduced-sodium tamari
1 tbsp poultry seasoning
1 tsp freshly ground black pepper
1 tbsp arrowroot powder
1 cup plain unsweetened almond milk
1 yellow onion, diced
2 cups low-sodium vegetable broth, divided
1 tbsp minced garlic
2 celery stalks, diced
40oz (1kg) mixed mushrooms, roughly chopped
½ cup dry white wine
2 cups chopped fresh spinach or other leafy greens
Chopped fresh flat-leaf parsley, to garnish
Smoked paprika or nutmeg, to garnish

1. To a blender, add the hemp seeds, nutritional yeast, lemon juice, apple cider vinegar, Worcestershire, tamari, poultry seasoning, pepper, arrowroot, and almond milk. Blend for 60 to 90 seconds until smooth and well combined. Set aside.

2. Heat a large saucepan or Dutch oven over medium-high heat. When hot, sauté the onion with as little broth as possible, just enough to avoid burning, for 3 minutes or until translucent. Add the garlic, and sauté for 30 to 60 seconds or until the garlic is lightly browned, being careful not to scorch. Add the celery, and cook for 2 minutes more, adding more broth as necessary, until soft.

3. Add the mushrooms, and cover. Allow the mushrooms to sweat until the pan is filled with liquid. (Watch carefully to avoid liquid spilling over.) They will reduce significantly. Uncover and allow some liquid to evaporate, about 3 to 5 minutes. Add the wine. Add the blended sauce and remaining broth, and bring to a boil. Reduce heat to low, and simmer for 10 to 15 minutes until thickened, stirring frequently. (You can add more broth to thin, if desired, as the soup will thicken significantly.) Add the spinach, and turn off the heat.

4. Garnish with parsley and a sprinkle of paprika or nutmeg. Enjoy immediately, or cool to room temperature and refrigerate in an airtight container for up to 5 days.

"Like Peas and Carrots" Soup

Prep Time: 20 minutes
Cook Time: 60 minutes
Serves: 4–6

"We was like peas and carrots," as per the movie *Forrest Gump*. This vegetable duo represents a perfect combination: the yin to the yang, the salt and pepper, the rice and beans. This recipe is a confluence of many trials with my dear friend Sharon, and we love its simplicity, vibrancy, and deliciousness.

For the carrot soup

1 shallot, chopped

2 cloves garlic, minced

3 cups thinly sliced carrots

½ cup chopped celery

1 cup peeled and diced potato

4 cups low-sodium vegetable broth

1 bay leaf

2 tsp ground coriander

½ tbsp miso paste

½ tsp freshly ground black pepper

1 tsp freshly squeezed lemon juice

1 cup plant milk

For the pea soup

1 shallot, chopped

1 clove garlic, minced

½ cup chopped celery

1 cup peeled and diced potato

4 cups low-sodium vegetable broth

1 (12oz; 340g) bag frozen peas

2 cups baby spinach

½ tbsp miso paste

½ tsp freshly ground black pepper

1 tsp freshly squeezed lemon juice

½ cup plant milk

1. To make the carrot soup, heat a large saucepan or Dutch oven over medium-high heat. When hot, sauté the shallot with as little water as possible, just enough to avoid burning, for 3 minutes or until translucent. Add the garlic, carrots, celery, and potato. Cook for 5 minutes more, adding water 1 tablespoon at a time as needed to avoid sticking.

2. Add the broth, bay leaf, and coriander; bring to a boil. When boiling, lower the heat to medium-low, and cook until the vegetables soften. Turn off the heat, and remove the bay leaf. Add the miso paste, and blend with an immersion blender. (Or transfer to a blender to purée.) Stir in the pepper, lemon juice, and plant milk; set aside.

3. To make the pea soup, heat another large saucepan or Dutch oven over medium-high heat. When hot, sauté the shallot with as little water as possible, just enough to avoid burning, for 3 minutes or until translucent. Add the garlic, celery, and potato. Cook for 5 minutes more, adding water 1 tablespoon at a time as needed to avoid sticking.

4. Add the broth, and bring to a boil. When boiling, lower the heat to medium, and simmer for 10 minutes or until the vegetables are soft. Add the peas, and bring back to a boil. Simmer for 5 minutes more. Add the spinach, and cook for 1 minute until wilted. Remove from the heat, stir in the miso paste, and blend with an immersion blender. (Or transfer to a blender to purée.) Stir in the pepper, lemon juice, and plant milk.

5. To make the duo, transfer the soups into separate pouring cups. Pour at the same time into a bowl, side by side. Feather the soups by using a fork to swirl down the middle, where the two soups converge. Enjoy hot, or store separately in airtight containers in the refrigerator for up to 5 days.

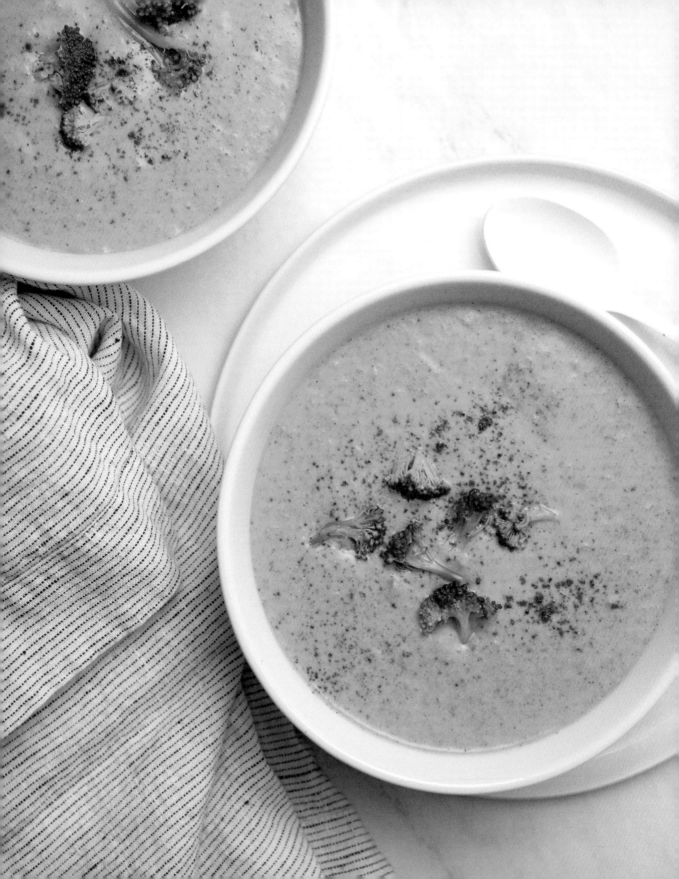

Nacho Broccoli Soup

Prep Time: 20 minutes
Cook Time: 50 minutes
Serves: 4

Na-cho broccoli soup—it's my broccoli soup! But I am always happy to share. This recipe is cheesy, spicy, ooey-gooey goodness in a pot. Making broccoli even better, butternut squash provides a smooth and starchy base for this sauce, which is made extra creamy with the addition of potato and cashews.

1 small butternut squash
1 Yukon Gold potato
1 (4oz; 113g) can green chiles
½ cup raw cashews
½ cup nutritional yeast
2 tbsp freshly squeezed lemon juice
1 tbsp low-sodium tamari
1 tbsp chili powder
1 tsp ground chipotle powder
½ tsp cayenne, plus more to garnish
2 cups plant milk
2 cups low-sodium vegetable broth
4 cups broccoli florets

1. Preheat the oven to 375°F (190°C). Line a baking sheet with parchment paper or a silicone baking mat. Place the butternut squash and potato on the baking sheet (whole) and roast until the skin of the squash is brown and bubbling, about 40 minutes.

2. When cool enough to handle, peel the squash, and remove the seeds. Measure out 2 cups cooked squash, and reserve any extra for another use. In a high-speed blender, combine the butternut squash, potato, chiles, cashews, nutritional yeast, lemon juice, tamari, chili powder, chipotle powder, cayenne, and plant milk. Blend on high until smooth and creamy.

3. In a medium saucepan, bring the broth to a boil over medium-high heat. Add the broccoli, and blanch for 2 to 4 minutes until the broccoli is bright green. With a slotted spoon, remove about 1 cup of the broccoli florets and set aside. Add the remaining broccoli and broth to the blender with the sauce. Blend until it reaches your desired consistency.

4. Serve hot, topped with the reserved broccoli florets and garnished with additional cayenne, if desired.

NOTE Hemp seeds can be substituted for cashews if there is an allergy or preference. And you can omit the cashews or seeds entirely, if desired.

One-Pot Staples Soup

Finally, a healthy recipe template that can be made in under 30 minutes using ingredients that are easy to keep stocked in your kitchen!

The premise here is that you can always have frozen vegetables in your freezer, as well as broth, canned tomatoes, beans, and spices in your pantry; so these recipes can be made quickly whenever you need something simple. Mix and match veggies, spices, and beans based on what you have. Whip up a batch, and you will have plenty to enjoy for days. Add a baked potato, cauliflower rice, or whole grain to plump up this meal.

Base Ingredients

1 (12oz; 340g) bag frozen chopped onion or 1 (10oz; 283g) pkg fresh chopped onion
3 (16oz; 450g) bags frozen vegetables (see flavor variations for vegetable suggestions)
4 cups low-sodium vegetable broth
2 tbsp reduced-sodium tamari
½–1 tsp freshly ground black pepper, to taste
½–1 tsp red pepper flakes
Fresh herbs (optional), to garnish
Sliced scallions (optional), to garnish

1. Heat a large saucepan or Dutch oven over medium-high heat. When hot, sauté the onion with as little broth as possible, just enough to avoid burning, for 3 minutes or until translucent.

2. Add the frozen mixed vegetables, tomatoes (if using), beans (if using), broth, pepper, red pepper flakes, and any other dried spices. Cover and bring to a boil.

3. When boiling, reduce the heat to low, and simmer for 10 to 20 minutes, stirring occasionally, until the vegetables are cooked through. Add the tamari and vinegar, if needed. Taste and adjust the seasonings. Remove the bay leaves, if using. Garnish with fresh herbs and sliced scallions, if desired, and serve hot.

4. Store in an airtight container in the refrigerator for up to 5 days.

flavor variations

Curry
Suggested veggies: cauliflower, carrots, peas, mushrooms, potatoes
1 (28oz; 794g) can crushed tomatoes (optional)
1 (15oz; 425g) can chickpeas (optional), drained and rinsed
2 bay leaves
1 tbsp curry powder
2 tbsp freshly squeezed lemon juice

Tex-Mex
Suggested veggies: bell peppers, corn, carrots, zucchini, green beans
1 (28oz; 794g) can crushed tomatoes (optional)
1 (15oz; 425g) can black or pinto beans (optional), drained and rinsed
2 bay leaves
1 tbsp chili powder
1 tsp ground cumin
1 tsp dried Mexican oregano
¼–½ tsp cayenne
1 tbsp freshly squeezed lime juice

Za'atar
Suggested veggies: cauliflower, hash brown/potatoes, peas,
    spinach, carrots, butternut squash, green beans
1 (28oz; 794g) can crushed tomatoes (optional)
1 (15oz; 425g) can chickpeas (optional), drained and rinsed
2 bay leaves
2 tbsp za'atar
2 tsp smoked paprika
1 tbsp balsamic vinegar or lemon juice

Italian
Suggested veggies: broccoli, zucchini, cauliflower, carrots,
    green beans, lima beans, peas, corn
1 (28oz; 794g) can crushed tomatoes (optional)
1 (15oz; 425g) can kidney beans (optional), drained and rinsed
2 bay leaves
1 tbsp Italian seasoning
1 tsp garlic powder
1 tbsp freshly squeezed lemon juice

Asian
Suggested veggies: stir-fry mixed vegetables, broccoli, carrots,
    cabbage, mushrooms
1 (15oz; 425g) pkg edamame (optional)
2 bay leaves
1 tbsp Chinese five spice powder
1 tsp ground ginger
1 tsp garlic powder
1 tbsp rice vinegar

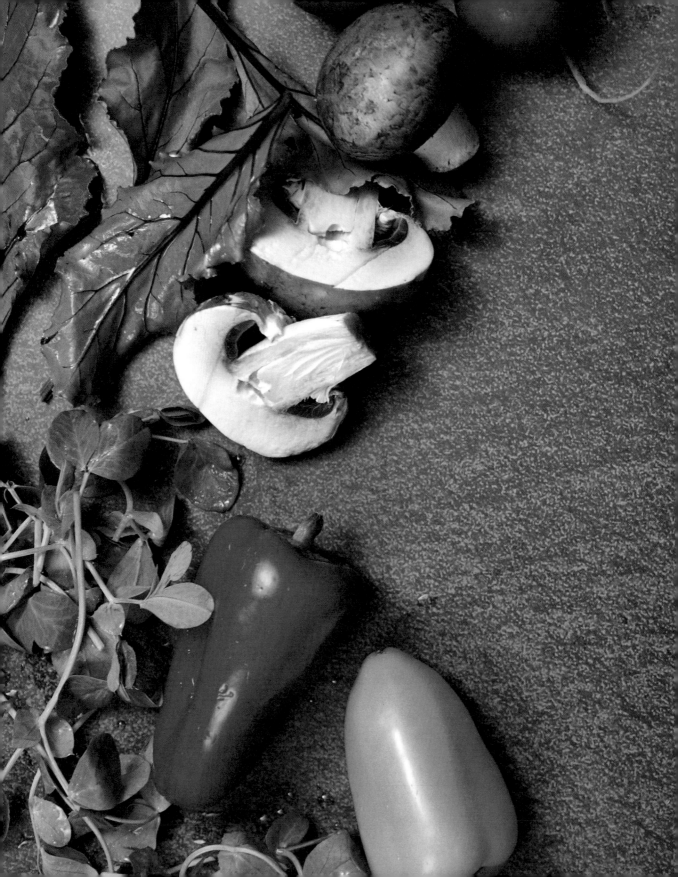

CHAPTER 7
PANS

Smoky Sweet Potato Mac 'n' Cheese

Prep Time: 5 minutes
Cook Time: 1 hour 15 minutes
Serves: 4

My two teenage kids would answer that age-old question, "What would you take with you if you were stranded on a deserted island?" with "Mac and cheese." Of course, this recipe is the "kid tested, mother approved," nutritious, delicious version that I would batch cook as much as possible for that island getaway.

2 medium sweet potatoes
½ cup raw cashews
4 tbsp nutritional yeast
1 tsp dry mustard powder
½ tsp garlic powder
½ tsp onion powder
½ tsp chipotle powder
½ tsp smoked paprika
2 tbsp freshly squeezed lemon juice
1 tbsp reduced-sodium tamari
2 cups plant milk
1 (8oz; 225g) pkg chickpea pasta shells or elbows
12oz (340g) broccoli florets
Freshly ground black pepper (optional), to serve

1. Preheat the oven to 400°F (200°C). Line a baking sheet with a silicone baking mat or parchment paper. Scrub the potatoes well and poke holes in the flesh a few times with a fork. Place on the prepared baking sheet, and bake for 40 to 60 minutes until juices begin to seep out and the potatoes are easily pierced with a toothpick or knife.

2. When cool, scoop the potato flesh from the skins and place in a high-powered blender. Add the cashews, nutritional yeast, mustard powder, garlic powder, onion powder, chipotle powder, paprika, lemon juice, tamari, and plant milk. Blend until smooth.

3. In a large saucepan, bring at least 8 cups water to a boil. Add the pasta and stir immediately. Cook to desired firmness, according to package directions, stirring occasionally. Add the broccoli, and cook for 1 to 2 minutes more until the broccoli is bright green. Drain, and return the pasta and broccoli to the saucepan. Add the cheesy sauce, reserving about 1 cup to drizzle on top, and stir to combine. Pour the mixture into a medium baking dish and top with the remaining cheesy sauce.

4. Broil on high for 5 to 10 minutes, until lightly browned on top. Serve hot, with pepper, if desired.

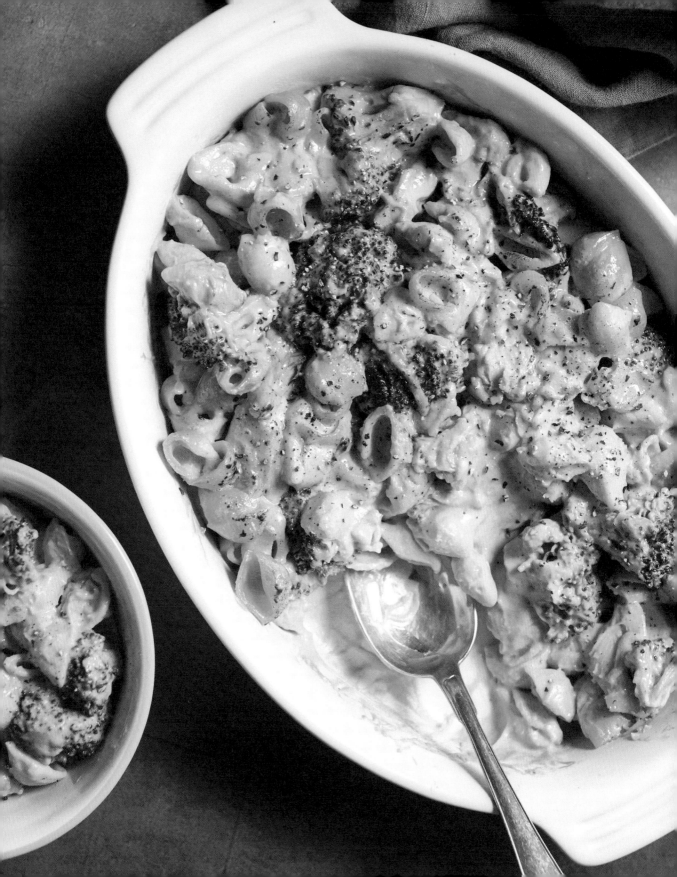

Prep Time: 10 minutes
Cook Time: 35 minutes
Serves: 2–4

Baba Ghanoushka

When the style of shakshuka meets the flavors of baba ghanoush, you get . . . baba ghanoushka! Instead of poached eggs dropped into a spicy, simmering tomato sauce, à la the traditional Middle Eastern breakfast dish, this version uses roasted eggplant.

1 medium eggplant, sliced into ½-in (1.25cm) rounds
2 tbsp tahini
1 tsp za'atar
1 yellow onion, finely chopped
1 red bell pepper, finely chopped
3 cloves garlic, minced
1½ tsp ground cumin
1 tsp smoked paprika
½ tsp red pepper flakes or harissa
¼ tsp freshly ground black pepper
1 (14.5oz; 411g) can fire-roasted crushed tomatoes
½ cup low-sodium vegetable broth
1 tbsp tomato paste
2 tbsp chopped fresh flat-leaf parsley, to garnish
Cooked or raw greens, to serve

1. Preheat the oven to 400°F (200°C). Line a baking sheet with parchment paper or a silicone baking mat.

2. Arrange the eggplant slices on the prepared baking sheet, spread evenly with tahini, and sprinkle with za'atar. Bake for 30 minutes or until browned.

3. Meanwhile, heat a large saucepan or Dutch oven over medium-high heat. When hot, sauté the onion with as little water as possible, just enough to avoid burning, for 3 minutes or until translucent. Add the bell pepper, and sauté over medium heat for 4 to 5 minutes or until it begins to soften, adding water as necessary to avoid burning. Add the garlic, cumin, paprika, red pepper flakes, and pepper. Cook for 1 minute more.

4. Add the tomatoes, broth, and tomato paste; increase the heat; and bring to a boil. When boiling, reduce the heat to medium, and simmer for 15 to 20 minutes until thickened.

5. Gently place the eggplant rounds on top of the sauce with tongs, and simmer for 5 minutes to allow the sauce to absorb into the rounds. Remove from the heat, garnish with parsley, and serve over cooked or raw greens.

Mashed Potato and Baked Bean Pie

Prep Time: 20 minutes
Cook Time: 1 hour 10 minutes
Serves: 4

While this dish takes a little time to prep, it is well worth the effort. Creamy, golden brown mashed potatoes, tomatoey beans, and umami-rich mushrooms with spinach, all in one large, satisfying, hearty baked pie. This is a super-shareable dish the whole family will enjoy, and it tastes even better the next day, once cooled and reheated.

4 medium russet potatoes, peeled and diced

½ yellow onion, diced

8oz (225g) cremini mushrooms, sliced

2 cloves garlic, minced

1 tbsp minced fresh thyme (or 1 tsp dried thyme)

2 tsp reduced-sodium tamari

1 tsp freshly ground black pepper, divided

2 cups packed baby spinach, chopped

2 tbsp yellow mustard

¼–½ cup plant milk

½ cup nutritional yeast, divided

1 (15oz; 425g) can cannellini beans, drained and rinsed

½ cup crushed tomatoes

2 tbsp tomato paste

2 tbsp ketchup

2 tbsp anchovy-free Worcestershire sauce

1. To a medium saucepan, add the potatoes and enough water to cover. Bring to a boil. When boiling, cover, reduce the heat to medium-low, and simmer for 15 minutes or until the potatoes are fork-tender.

2. Meanwhile, heat a medium saucepan over medium-high heat. When hot, sauté the onion with as little water as possible, just enough to avoid burning, for 3 minutes or until translucent. Add the mushrooms, garlic, and thyme. Cover, and allow the mushrooms to release their liquid. Remove the lid, and continue to cook for 5 minutes or until the liquid cooks off. Add the tamari and ½ teaspoon black pepper. Turn off the heat, and stir in the spinach. Allow the spinach to wilt, stirring frequently. Remove from the heat, and set aside.

3. Preheat the oven to 400°F (200°C). Drain the cooked potatoes, and transfer to a large bowl. Add the mustard, plant milk, and ¼ cup nutritional yeast, as well as the remaining ½ teaspoon black pepper. Mash until smooth. The mixture should be sticky and not too moist. If the mixture is too dry, add plant milk, 1 tablespoon at a time, until sticky and smooth.

4. In a medium bowl, combine the beans, tomatoes, tomato paste, ketchup, Worcestershire, and the remaining ¼ cup nutritional yeast. Toss to combine.

5. In a 9-inch (23cm) square baking dish or deep-dish pie pan, spread about two-thirds of the mashed potato mixture, using a spatula to press it into the bottom and up the sides of the pan, creating a well in the center for the remaining ingredients. Cover with the bean mixture, followed by the spinach and mushrooms. Spread the remaining mashed potatoes on top, making sure to cover all of the other ingredients. Bake for 45 minutes, and serve hot.

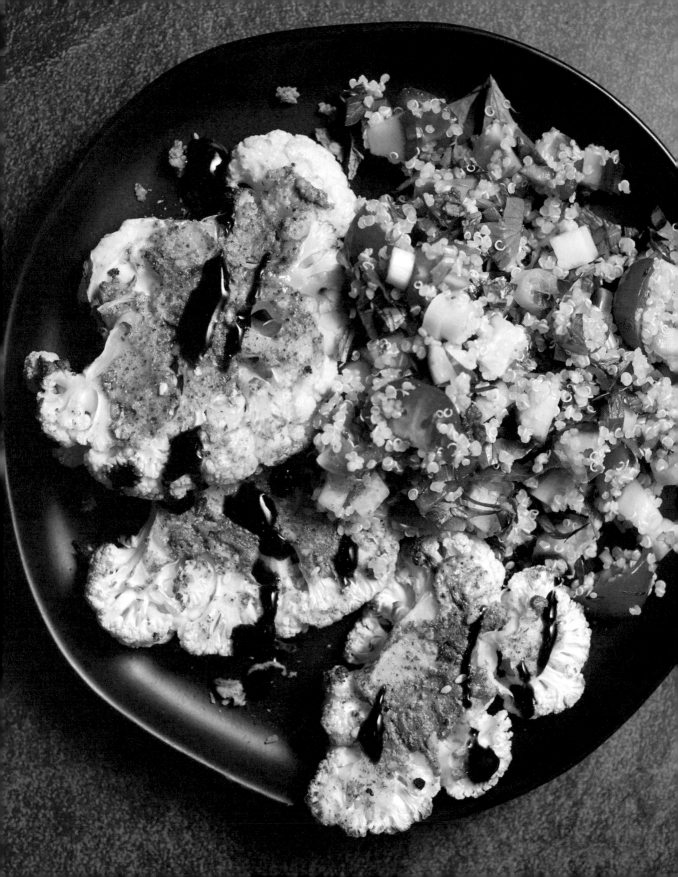

Tahini Za'atar Cauliflower Steaks
with Quinoa Tabbouleh

Prep Time: 30 minutes
Cook Time: 50 minutes
Serves: 2–4

Yet another delicious way to enjoy cauliflower—make it the center of your plate. Featuring flavors of the Middle East, this pairing of roasted cauliflower "steaks" with fresh and vibrant tabbouleh is well rounded and fulfilling.

2 tbsp tahini

2 tsp za'atar

2 tsp freshly squeezed lemon juice

2 tsp water, plus more as needed

1 head cauliflower, cut into ¾-in (2cm) steaks

Balsamic glaze (optional), to garnish

For the tabbouleh

½ cup quinoa, rinsed

¾ cup water

1 cup finely chopped cucumber

1 cup finely chopped fresh tomatoes

½ cup finely chopped fresh flat-leaf parsley, packed

½ cup finely chopped fresh mint, packed

¼ cup sliced scallions

3 tbsp freshly squeezed lemon juice

1 clove garlic, minced

1. To make the tabbouleh, place the quinoa in a small saucepan over medium-high heat, stirring until the excess water evaporates and the quinoa begins to toast. Add the water, cover with a lid, and bring to a boil over high heat. When boiling, cover, reduce heat to low, and simmer for 15 minutes. Remove from the heat with the lid still on, and allow to steam for 10 minutes. Transfer the cooked quinoa to a large bowl, and set aside to cool.

2. Meanwhile, preheat the oven to 450°F (230°C), and line a baking sheet with parchment paper or a silicone baking mat. To a small bowl, add the tahini, za'atar, lemon juice, and water, adding more water if needed to create a spreadable paste.

3. Place the cauliflower steaks on the prepared baking sheet. Coat one side of the cauliflower with a thin layer of the tahini paste, reserving half of the total mixture. Bake for 20 minutes. Carefully flip the cauliflower over, and spread the remaining paste on the opposite side. Bake for 10 minutes more or until golden brown.

4. To the cooled quinoa, add the cucumber, tomatoes, parsley, mint, scallions, lemon juice, and garlic; toss to combine. Serve the tabbouleh with the cauliflower steaks. Garnish with a drizzle of balsamic glaze, if desired.

> **NOTE** When preparing the cauliflower, some florets will naturally fall off as the center of the cauliflower head becomes the steaks. Include those florets in the process for extra bites.

Prep Time: 15 minutes + preparing croutons

Cook Time: 15 minutes

Serves: 2

Creole Tofu Scramble

Tofu scrambles are a fun and tasty way to enjoy soy, a versatile legume that is loaded with calcium, iron, and omega-3 fatty acids. Creole cuisine draws on several different cultures that offer unique flavors, providing this scramble with a spicy twist. Creole seasoning blends are easy to find, but they typically contain salt. Use this basic recipe, or look for a salt-free version.

½ red onion, chopped

½ green bell pepper, chopped

2 cloves garlic, minced

1 cup chopped cremini mushrooms

1 (16oz; 450g) pkg extra-firm tofu, crumbled

½ tsp ground turmeric

2 tsp Creole Seasoning Blend (see note)

¼ cup plant milk

4 tbsp nutritional yeast

1 tbsp reduced-sodium tamari

1 large tomato, chopped

2 cups chopped baby kale or spinach

3 tbsp chopped fresh flat-leaf parsley

1 tsp freshly ground black pepper, to taste

1 batch **Potato Croutons** (page 92)

Hot sauce (optional), to serve

1. Heat a large saucepan or Dutch oven over medium-high heat. Dry sauté the onion and bell pepper with as little water as possible, just enough to avoid burning, for 3 minutes or until the onion is translucent. Add the garlic, and cook for 30 seconds. Add the mushrooms, and cook for 5 minutes until the mushrooms have released their liquid, adding water as necessary to avoid sticking.

2. Add the tofu, turmeric, and Creole Seasoning Blend; stir to combine. Stir in the plant milk, nutritional yeast, and tamari; cook for 2 minutes until the liquid is absorbed. Add the tomato, and cook for another 2 minutes. Add the kale, parsley, and pepper; cook until the kale is wilted. Serve immediately with potato croutons and hot sauce, if desired.

> NOTE To make **Creole Seasoning Blend,** in a small bowl, mix together the following: 2 ½ tbsp paprika, 2 tbsp garlic powder, 1 tbsp freshly ground black pepper, 1 tbsp onion powder, 1 tbsp cayenne (reduce or replace with chili powder for less heat), 1 tbsp dried oregano, 1 tbsp dried thyme. Transfer to an airtight jar for storage.

Spicy Chickpea Loaf

Prep Time: 20 minutes + 1 hour to set
Cook Time: 1 hour 5 minutes
Serves: 6

A loaf is a traditional dish in the American kitchen, as well as throughout other parts of the world. This classic comfort food is usually made with meat, but here, chickpeas take center stage. Because this is a hearty, concentrated pan of wholesome goodness, it is a perfect recipe to whip up on a Sunday and enjoy throughout the week, volumized with side dishes.

1 small yellow onion, chopped
3–4 cloves garlic, minced
1 red bell pepper, chopped
1 cup chopped celery
2 (15oz; 425g) cans chickpeas
4 tbsp nutritional yeast
2 tbsp reduced-sodium tamari
1 tbsp tahini
1 tbsp tomato paste
1 tbsp Dijon mustard
1 tbsp balsamic vinegar
1 tbsp anchovy-free Worcestershire sauce
1 tbsp poultry seasoning
½ tsp freshly ground black pepper
2 cups rolled oats
¼ cup sriracha
1 tbsp date syrup or molasses
Cooked or raw greens (optional), to serve

1. Heat a large saucepan or Dutch oven over medium-high heat. When hot, sauté the onion with as little water as possible, just enough to avoid burning, for 3 minutes or until translucent. Add the garlic, and cook for 1 minute more, adding 1 tablespoon water, if needed. Add the bell pepper and celery, and sauté over medium heat for 4 to 5 minutes until the vegetables soften, adding water as necessary to avoid burning. Remove from the heat.

2. Drain the chickpeas, reserving ¼ cup aquafaba (liquid from can). In a food processor, combine the chickpeas, reserved aquafaba, sautéed vegetables, nutritional yeast, tamari, tahini, tomato paste, mustard, balsamic vinegar, Worcestershire, poultry seasoning, and pepper. Process until smooth, stopping to scrape the sides of the bowl once or twice. Pulse in the oats until well combined.

3. Transfer the mixture to an 8-inch (20cm) loaf pan (silicone, if possible, or lined with parchment paper), cover with foil, and place in the refrigerator for at least 1 hour to set.

4. Preheat oven to 375°F (190°C). In a small bowl, combine the sriracha and date syrup. Spread evenly over the loaf and cover with foil. Bake for 40 minutes. Remove the foil, and bake for 15 minutes more. Serve hot over a bed of cooked or raw greens, if desired.

NOTE This is a calorie-dense dish, so eat a smaller portion along with steamed or roasted veggies—such as broccoli, cauliflower, or kale—or serve with a raw green salad with balsamic vinegar dressing.

Prep Time: 20 minutes
Cook Time: 50 minutes
Serves: 4

Autumnal Stuffed Mushrooms

These munchable mushrooms offer several of the most nutritious and satisfying foods for weight loss all in one dish. Cruciferous goodness times two, mushroom magnificence, plus a daily dose of omega-3 fatty acid–rich hemp seeds. Enjoy these as an appetizer with guests or as a main meal over a bed of greens. Top with a drizzle of balsamic glaze or, if you are feeling ambitious, try the bright and vibrant cranberry gastrique option.

4 cups cauliflower florets or 1 (16oz; 450g) pkg cauliflower rice
½ cup hemp seeds
4 tbsp nutritional yeast
1 tbsp poultry seasoning
1 tbsp arrowroot powder
1 tbsp freshly squeezed lemon juice
1 tbsp apple cider vinegar
1 tbsp anchovy-free Worcestershire sauce
1 tbsp reduced-sodium tamari
¼–½ tsp red pepper flakes
¼–½ tsp freshly ground black pepper
2 cups plant milk
1 yellow onion, diced
2–4 celery stalks, diced
1 jalapeño, deseeded and finely diced
1 tbsp minced garlic
2 cups chopped kale

24 cremini mushrooms, stems removed
Arugula (optional), to serve
Balsamic glaze (optional), to serve

For the cranberry gastrique (optional)
¼ cup maple syrup
¼ cup apple cider vinegar
¾ cup fresh or frozen cranberries

1. In a food processor, pulse the cauliflower florets into rice. You may need to work in batches, depending on the size of your food processor. (Alternatively, you can use prericed cauliflower and skip this step.)

2. To a high-speed blender, add the hemp seeds, nutritional yeast, poultry seasoning, arrowroot, lemon juice, apple cider vinegar, Worcestershire, tamari, red pepper flakes, black pepper, and plant milk. Blend for 60 to 90 seconds until smooth and well combined. Set aside.

3. Heat a large saucepan or Dutch oven over medium-high heat. When hot, sauté the onion with as little water as possible, just enough to avoid burning, for 3 to 4 minutes or until it begins to brown. Add the celery and jalapeño, and continue to cook, adding water as necessary to prevent sticking, for 2 minutes or until soft. Add the garlic, and sauté for another 30 to 60 seconds or until lightly browned.

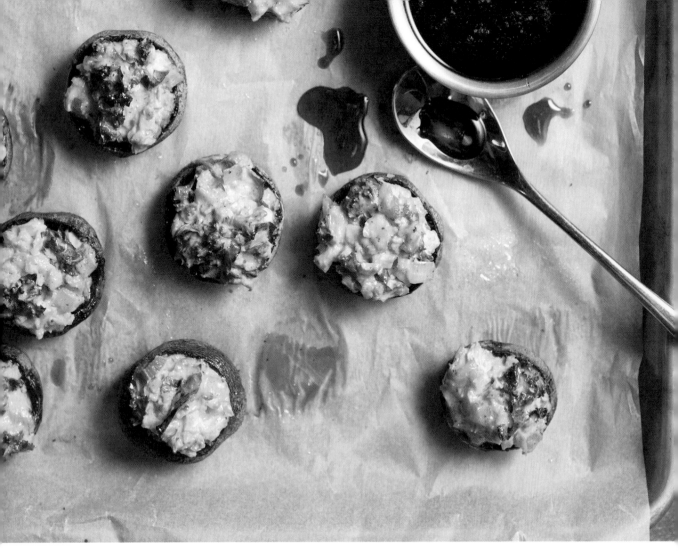

4. Add the cauliflower rice and blended sauce to the pan, and stir to combine. Reduce the heat to medium-low, and cook for 20 minutes until thickened, stirring frequently. Add the kale, and stir until wilted. Remove from the heat.

5. Preheat the oven to 350°F (175°C). Line a baking sheet with parchment paper. Place the mushroom caps on the prepared baking sheet. Fill each mushroom cap with the cauliflower rice mixture. (If there is leftover filling, refrigerate in an airtight container for up to 5 days.)

6. Bake for 25 to 30 minutes or until the filling is firm and golden and the mushrooms have released most of their liquid.

7. To make the optional cranberry gastrique, in a small saucepan over medium-high heat, heat the maple syrup, apple cider vinegar, and cranberries. When boiling, reduce the heat to medium-low, and simmer until the berries burst and the sauce reduces.

8. Serve the mushrooms on a bed of arugula with a drizzle of balsamic glaze or the cranberry gastrique, if desired.

Prep Time: 15 minutes

Cook Time: 40 minutes

Serves: 2

Simple Spaghetti Squash Caulifredo

Nutrify your Alfredo sauce with cruciferous cauliflower rice and cashews, and pour it over the always lovely spaghetti squash for a treat that mimics a classic pasta Alfredo without all of the calories. This sauce can also be enjoyed with zucchini noodles ("zoodles") or butternut squash noodles, or served over steamed vegetables or baked potatoes. It is quick and easy to blend up, so try experimenting with your favorite combinations.

1 medium spaghetti squash

Fresh basil or flat-leaf parsley (optional), to garnish

For the sauce

12oz (340g) frozen cauliflower rice

¼ cup raw cashews

2 cloves garlic, minced

¼ cup nutritional yeast

1 tbsp reduced-sodium tamari

1 tbsp freshly squeezed lemon juice

½ tsp onion powder

¼ tsp freshly ground black pepper

⅛ tsp ground nutmeg

½ cup plant milk

1. Preheat the oven to 375°F (190°C). Line a baking sheet with parchment paper or a silicone baking mat. Cut the spaghetti squash in half lengthwise (see note), and remove the seeds with a spoon. Place the squash cut side down on the prepared baking sheet. Bake for 40 minutes until lightly browned on the outside. Remove from the oven, and set aside to cool.

2. Meanwhile, to make the sauce, heat the cauliflower rice according to the package instructions. To a blender, add the cauliflower rice, cashews, garlic, nutritional yeast, tamari, lemon juice, onion powder, pepper, nutmeg, and plant milk. Blend until smooth.

3. When the squash is cool enough to handle, scrape out the flesh with a fork to create spaghetti-like strands. Place the spaghetti squash strands in a serving bowl, pour the sauce over top, and toss to combine. Garnish with basil or parsley, if using, and serve warm.

> **NOTE** To soften the exterior of the squash and make it easier to cut, microwave whole spaghetti squash for a few minutes prior to cutting.

Rich Lentil Ragu

Prep Time: 20 minutes
Cook Time: 50–60 minutes
Serves: 4–6

Classic *ragu* is an Italian meat-based sauce served over pasta. In this recipe, lentils lend texture and, together with the vegetables, create a rich, nutritious sauce loaded with umami goodness. Make a batch (or two) to eat throughout the week. Enjoy on its own, or serve over spaghetti squash, steamed broccolini, polenta, or a baked potato for a hearty, satisfying meal.

1 yellow onion, diced
2 carrots, finely diced
3 celery stalks, finely diced
1 cup finely diced mushrooms
1 red bell pepper, diced
4 cups low-sodium vegetable broth, divided
3 cloves garlic, minced
1 tsp dried thyme
1 tsp dried oregano
¼ cup finely chopped sun-dried tomatoes (not packed in oil)
¼–½ tsp red pepper flakes
½ cup red wine or vegetable broth
1 cup green lentils, rinsed
2 bay leaves
2 cups crushed tomatoes
2 tbsp tomato paste

1 tbsp balsamic vinegar
1 tbsp reduced-sodium tamari
1 tsp freshly ground black pepper or more, to taste
2 cups chopped baby spinach
Fresh basil (optional), to serve
Nutritional yeast (optional), to serve

1. Heat a large saucepan or Dutch oven over medium-high heat. When hot, sauté the onion with as little water as possible, just enough to avoid burning, for 3 minutes or until translucent. Add the carrot, celery, mushrooms, bell pepper, and ¼ cup broth. Cook for 6 to 8 minutes, stirring frequently.

2. Add the garlic, thyme, oregano, sun-dried tomatoes, and red pepper flakes; cook for 1 minute. Stir in the wine, and cook for 2 to 3 minutes or until the liquid evaporates. Add the lentils, bay leaves, remaining 3 ¾ cups broth, crushed tomatoes, and tomato paste. Bring to a boil, lower the heat, and simmer for 40 minutes or until the lentils are soft.

3. Remove the bay leaves, and stir in the vinegar, tamari, black pepper, and spinach. Stir, and turn off the heat once the spinach is wilted. Garnish with fresh basil and a sprinkle of nutritional yeast, if desired.

Potato Croutons

This is the best thing to happen since sliced bread. Literally. Batch cook potatoes, and keep them in the fridge so you can make these—in any and every flavor profile—anytime. You add nutrition, flavor, and fun by including these clever croutons in plates, pots, pans, and power bowls or enjoying them their own. Double, triple, or quadruple this recipe—add them everywhere.

1 medium russet potato, peeled and cut into crouton-sized pieces
Seasoning blend of choice

1. To a medium saucepan, add the potatoes and enough water to cover. Cover with a lid, and bring to a boil over medium-high heat. When boiling, reduce the heat, and simmer until the potatoes are fork-tender, about 10 to 15 minutes, depending on the size. Drain, and set aside to cool.

2. Preheat the oven to 450°F (230°C). Line a baking sheet with parchment paper or a silicone baking mat. In a medium bowl, combine all ingredients for your seasoning blend of choice. Add the potatoes, and toss to coat with seasonings.

3. Spread the seasoned potatoes evenly on the prepared baking sheet. Bake until crispy, about 40 to 45 minutes, depending on the size of the croutons. Toss midway for even browning.

seasoning blends

Asian
1 tsp sesame seeds
1 tsp garlic powder
1 tsp onion powder
½ tsp ground ginger
½ tsp red pepper flakes
   (optional)

Rye
2 tsp caraway seeds
1 tsp garlic powder
1 tsp onion powder
½ tsp freshly ground
   black pepper
1 tbsp nutritional yeast
   (optional)

Curry
1 tsp curry powder
½ tsp ground turmeric
½ tsp freshly ground
   black pepper
1 tbsp nutritional yeast
   (optional)

Cheesy Rosemary
2 tsp dried rosemary
1 tbsp nutritional yeast
1 tsp garlic powder
1 tsp onion powder
½ tsp freshly ground
   black pepper

Za'atar
2 tsp za'atar
1 tbsp nutritional yeast
   (optional)

Ranch
1 tbsp nutritional yeast
1 tsp dried dill
1 tsp dried parsley
1 tsp garlic powder
1 tsp onion powder
½ tsp freshly ground
   black pepper
1 tbsp apple cider or
   white vinegar

Prep Time: 15 minutes +
preparing sauce
Cook Time: 1 hour 40 minutes
Serves: 3–4

Spaghetti (Squash) Lasagna

Here's a noodle-free, nutrient-dense, simple lasagna that will impress your friends and family. As someone who is intimidated by cutting squash, I was thrilled to learn that you can microwave the squash for a few minutes first to make cutting it easier and safer, opening up a whole new world of possibilities.

2 medium spaghetti squash
1 batch **Simple Marinara Sauce** (page 162)
1 tbsp nutritional yeast
1–3 tsp red pepper flakes (optional)

For the tofu ricotta
1 (16oz; 450g) pkg extra-firm tofu, crumbled
3 tbsp nutritional yeast
2 tbsp freshly squeezed lemon juice
1 tbsp red wine vinegar
1 tsp dried basil
1 tsp dried oregano
1 tsp dried rosemary

For the cashew drizzle
½ cup raw cashews
3 tbsp nutritional yeast
1 tsp onion powder
1 tsp garlic powder
1 tsp freshly squeezed lemon juice
½ cup plant milk

1. Preheat the oven to 375°F (190°C). Line a baking sheet with parchment paper or a silicone baking mat.

2. Cut the squash in half lengthwise, and remove the seeds with a spoon. (You can microwave whole spaghetti squash for a few minutes prior to cutting to soften the exterior and make it easier to cut.) Place the squash cut side down on the prepared baking sheet. Bake for 40 minutes until lightly browned on the outside. Remove from the oven, and set aside to cool.

3. Meanwhile, prepare the tofu ricotta. In a large bowl, combine the tofu, nutritional yeast, lemon juice, red wine vinegar, basil, oregano, and rosemary. Mix well, and set aside.

4. To make the cashew drizzle, combine all ingredients in a high-speed blender. Blend until smooth, and set aside.

5. Using a fork, scrape the flesh from the cooled squash into a bowl, creating spaghetti-like strands.

6. Spread half of the marinara sauce in a 9 × 13-inch (23 × 33cm) baking dish, followed by half the squash, all of the tofu ricotta, the remaining squash, and the remaining marinara sauce. Finally, top with the cashew drizzle. Sprinkle with nutritional yeast and some red pepper flakes, if desired. Cover with foil, and bake for 30 minutes. Remove the foil, and bake for 20 to 30 minutes more. Serve hot.

Green Beans with Potatoes

Prep Time: 10 minutes
Cook Time: 25 minutes
Serves: 4

A hearty, simple, satisfying stew of velvety potatoes; tender green beans; and bright, lemony tomatoes with earthy undertones of turmeric and cumin.

1 medium yellow onion, chopped
2 cloves garlic, minced
3 cups Yukon Gold or russet potatoes, chopped
1 (16oz; 450g) bag frozen green beans
1 tbsp ground turmeric
1 tsp ground cumin
½ tsp freshly ground black pepper
½ tsp red pepper flakes
1 (14.5oz; 411g) can crushed tomatoes
1 cup low-sodium vegetable broth
1 tbsp freshly squeezed lemon juice
½ tsp maple syrup
½ cup chopped fresh parsley, to garnish

1. Heat a large saucepan or Dutch oven over medium-high heat. When hot, sauté the onion with as little water as possible, just enough to avoid burning, for 3 minutes or until translucent and beginning to caramelize.

2. Add the garlic, and cook for 30 to 45 seconds until golden brown. Add the potatoes, green beans, turmeric, cumin, black pepper, red pepper flakes, tomatoes, and broth. Bring to a boil over medium-high heat. When boiling, cover, and lower heat to medium. Simmer for 15 minutes, stirring occasionally, until the potatoes are soft.

3. Stir in the lemon juice and maple syrup, cover, and simmer for 5 minutes. Garnish with parsley and serve immediately, or store in an airtight container in the refrigerator for up to 5 days.

Prep Time: 30 minutes
Cook Time: 60 minutes
Serves: 4

Chick-less Pot Pie

All the indulgence of a timeless classic, but healthy enough to be in regular rotation on your menu. If you prefer to skip the soy curls, add an additional can of chickpeas or try using mushrooms or baked tofu instead.

1 cup dried soy curls (optional, but recommended)

2 large russet potatoes, sliced thinly into circles (using a mandoline, if possible)

3¼ cups low-sodium vegetable broth, divided

1 yellow onion, chopped

2 cloves garlic, minced

2 carrots, chopped

2 celery stalks, chopped

1 red bell pepper, chopped

1 cup chopped green beans (fresh or frozen)

1 cup peas (fresh or frozen)

1 (15oz; 425g) can chickpeas, drained and rinsed

1 cup plant milk

1 bay leaf

1 tbsp poultry seasoning

1 tbsp anchovy-free Worcestershire sauce

1 tsp freshly ground black pepper

2 tbsp arrowroot powder

1 tbsp miso paste

1 tbsp freshly squeezed lemon juice

½ cup chopped fresh flat-leaf parsley

1. In a medium bowl, rehydrate the soy curls, if using, in water.

2. To a medium saucepan, add the potatoes and 3 cups broth. Bring to a boil over medium-high heat. Once boiling, lower the heat, and simmer for 5 minutes or until the potatoes are pliable. Remove from the heat and drain, reserving the broth used for cooking. Set aside.

3. Preheat the oven to 425°F (220°C). Heat a large saucepan or Dutch oven over medium-high heat. When hot, sauté the onion with as little water as possible, just enough to avoid burning, for 3 minutes or until translucent. Add the garlic, and sauté for 1 minute more. Add the carrot, celery, and bell pepper. Cook for 4 to 5 minutes until softened, adding a few tablespoons of water if needed to avoid burning.

4. Squeeze any excess water from the soy curls, and cut them into bite-sized pieces. Add the soy curls, green beans, and peas to the pan, and sauté until any excess liquid is absorbed.

5. Add the reserved broth from cooking the potatoes along with the chickpeas, plant milk, bay leaf, poultry seasoning, Worcestershire, and pepper. Bring to a boil. When boiling, reduce the heat to a simmer.

6. In a small bowl, whisk the remaining ¼ cup broth with the arrowroot to make a slurry. Add the slurry to the pan, and simmer for 5 to 10 minutes until the mixture has thickened.

7. In small bowl, combine the miso paste with a few tablespoons of hot broth from the pan and stir to dissolve. Add the dissolved miso paste, lemon juice, and parsley to the pan, and stir. Remove the bay leaf, and remove from the heat.

8. Pour the mixture into a 9 × 13-inch (23 × 33cm) baking dish. Layer the sliced potatoes on top in even rows. Bake for 30 to 40 minutes until the potatoes brown and crisp up. Serve hot.

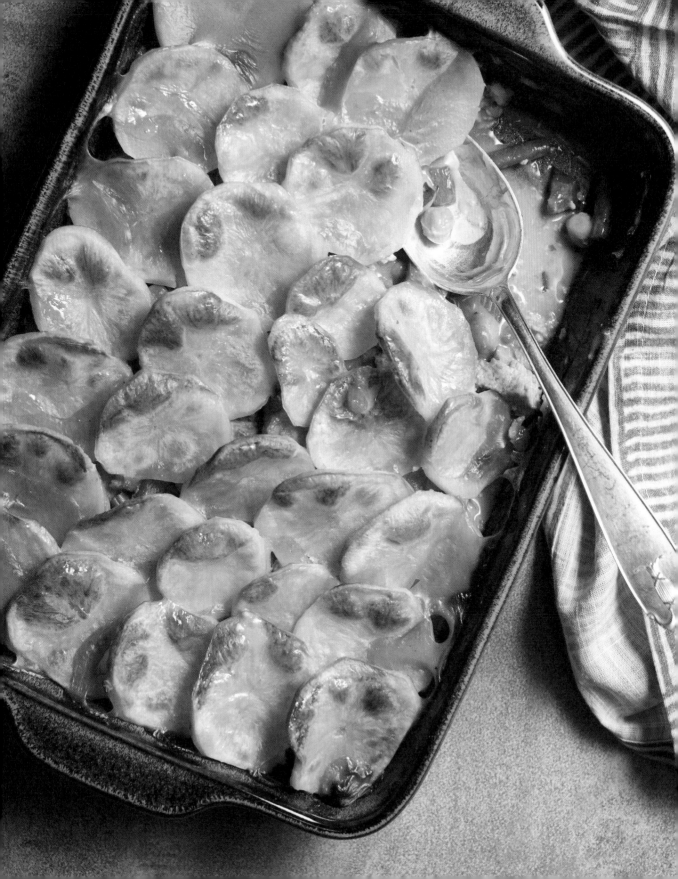

Prep Time: 30 minutes + 1 hour to marinate
Cook Time: 20 minutes
Serves: 2–4

Saag Paneer

One of my all-time favorite dishes is this Indian curry, and when I went plant-based, I missed the special texture that the paneer (a cheese) offered. Marinating tofu in cashew cream is a game changer. Fenugreek leaves may be tricky to find, but they can be purchased in specialty stores or ordered online. Their flavor makes the dish unique, and a bag will last a while.

½ cup raw cashews
¼ cup nutritional yeast
1 cup plant milk
1 (16oz; 450g) pkg extra-firm tofu, pressed, blotted dry, and cut into cubes
1lb (450g) baby spinach
1 medium jalapeño, deseeded and roughly chopped
1-in (2.5cm) piece fresh ginger, minced or roughly chopped
1 tbsp cumin seeds
1 white or yellow onion, diced
1 tsp ground cumin
1 tsp ground coriander
¼ tsp ground turmeric
4 cloves garlic, minced
1 cup chopped tomatoes
2 tsp garam masala
2 tsp dried fenugreek leaves
½ cup chopped fresh cilantro (optional), to garnish

1. To a high-speed blender, add the cashews, nutritional yeast, and plant milk. Blend until smooth. To a medium food-storage container, add the cubed tofu. Pour the cashew cream over the tofu, and toss gently to coat, taking care not to smash the cubes. Place in the refrigerator to marinate for at least 1 hour or overnight, if possible.

2. Preheat the oven to 400°F (200°C). Line a baking sheet with parchment paper or a silicone baking mat. In a medium saucepan, bring 4 cups water to a boil. While the water comes to a boil, prepare an ice bath. When boiling, quickly blanch the spinach until just wilted, 1 to 2 minutes, before the color changes from bright green. Drain well, and place in the ice bath to cool. When cool, press with a clean cloth, nut bag, or potato ricer to remove as much water as possible.

3. Carefully remove the tofu cubes from the cashew cream marinade, and place on the prepared baking sheet. Bake for 15 minutes or until golden brown. Set aside. To a high-speed blender, add the reserved cashew cream (used to marinate tofu), cooked spinach, jalapeño, ginger, and 1 to 2 tablespoons water. Blend until smooth.

4. Heat a medium saucepan over medium-high heat. Add the cumin seeds, and toast for 1 minute until fragrant. Add the onion along with 1 to 2 tablespoons water, just enough to avoid burning. Cook until lightly browned, adding water as needed to prevent burning. Add the ground cumin, coriander, and turmeric. Cook for 1 minute or until fragrant. Add the garlic, and cook for 30 seconds, stirring frequently.

5. Reduce the heat, add the tomatoes, and cook for 10 minutes or until the tomatoes soften. Add the spinach sauce, and simmer for 2 minutes. Stir in the garam masala and fenugreek leaves. Gently place the tofu into the pan, and simmer until the tofu is just warmed through. Stir in the cilantro, if using, and serve hot.

Mexican Cauliflower Rice

Prep Time: 10–15 minutes
Cook Time: 20 minutes
Serves: 2–4

This dish is a colorful festival of flavors and ingredients, amped up in nutrition with cruciferous cauliflower as its base and kale wilted in at the end. Top this with Nacho Squash Sauce (page 165) or Sweet Potato Cheesy Sauce (page 163) for an extra-special treat.

4 cups cauliflower florets or 1 (16oz; 450g) pkg cauliflower rice

1 cup diced yellow onion

3 cloves garlic, minced

¼ cup minced jalapeño

1 cup frozen corn kernels

1 (15oz; 425g) can black beans, drained and rinsed

1 (15oz; 425g) can diced tomatoes

2 tbsp tomato paste

2 tbsp chili powder

1 tsp ground cumin

1 tsp dried oregano

1 tsp smoked paprika

½–1 tsp ground chipotle powder

2 cups finely chopped kale

1 cup chopped fresh cilantro, loosely packed

2 tsp freshly squeezed lime juice

1 tsp reduced-sodium tamari

1 tsp liquid smoke (optional)

1 tbsp nutritional yeast (optional), to garnish

Sliced scallions (optional), to garnish

1. In a food processor, pulse the cauliflower florets into rice. You may need to work in batches, depending on the container size. (Skip this step if using prericed cauliflower.)

2. Heat a large saucepan or Dutch oven over medium-high heat. When hot, sauté the onion with as little water as possible, just enough to avoid burning, for 3 to 4 minutes or until it begins to brown. Add the garlic and sauté for 30 to 60 seconds or until the garlic is lightly browned, being careful not to scorch.

3. Add the jalapeño with a splash of additional water, if needed. Cook for 1 to 2 minutes. Add the corn and beans, and stir. Add the cauliflower rice, tomatoes, tomato paste, chili powder, cumin, oregano, paprika, and chipotle powder. Stir to combine. Cover and simmer for 6 to 8 minutes until the cauliflower is cooked through and the liquid has thickened.

4. Add the kale, cover, and simmer for 3 to 4 minutes more until the kale is wilted. Add the cilantro, lime juice, tamari, and liquid smoke, if using. Toss to combine, and remove from the heat. Serve warm, garnished with nutritional yeast and scallions, if desired.

> NOTE This colorful cauliflower rice can be used as the filling for Tex-Mex Stuffed Peppers (page 123).

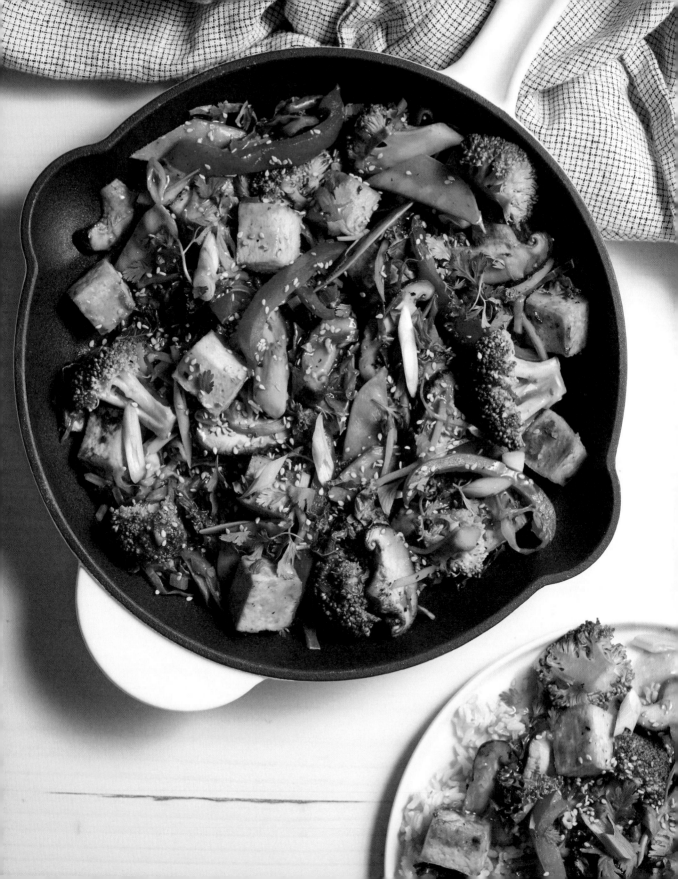

"Strong Bone" Stir-Fry

Prep Time: 10 minutes
Cook Time: 40 minutes
Serves: 2

This recipe demonstrates a delicious way to incorporate foods on a plant-based diet that promote bone health. Broccoli, cabbage, kale, and tofu are high in calcium. Tofu is also rich in isoflavones, which are associated with bone strengthening. Vitamin K, a crucial nutrient in bone health, is found in its optimal, low-oxalate version from the cabbage, kale, and bok choy.

1 (12oz; 340g) pkg extra-firm tofu, cubed
1 shallot, chopped
2 cloves garlic, minced
2 tsp minced fresh ginger
1 (8oz; 225g) package shiitake or cremini mushrooms, sliced
½ cup shredded carrots
1 red bell pepper, sliced
½ cup snow peas, sliced
½ cup shredded purple cabbage
2 cups broccoli florets
2 cups sliced kale
1 baby bok choy, sliced
Cooked cauliflower rice, brown rice, or quinoa (optional), to serve
1 tbsp sesame seeds
¼ cup sliced scallions
¼ cup chopped fresh cilantro

For the sauce
1 cup low-sodium vegetable broth
2 tbsp rice wine vinegar
2 tbsp sweet chili sauce
1 tbsp reduced-sodium tamari
1–2 tbsp sriracha, to taste
1½ tsp cornstarch

1. Preheat the oven to 400°F (200°C). Line a baking sheet with parchment paper or a silicone baking mat. Place the tofu cubes on the prepared baking sheet. Bake for 20 minutes, flip, and bake for 10 to 15 minutes more until browned. Set aside.

2. To make the sauce, in a small saucepan, combine the broth, rice wine vinegar, sweet chili sauce, tamari, and sriracha. Bring to a boil over medium-high heat. When boiling, reduce the heat, and stir in the cornstarch. Cook, stirring constantly, for 5 minutes or until thickened. Remove from the heat.

3. Heat a large wok or skillet over medium-high heat. When hot, sauté the shallot with as little water as possible, just enough to avoid burning, for 3 minutes until browned. Add the garlic and ginger, and stir for 1 minute, adding water as needed to avoid burning. Add the mushrooms, carrots, and bell pepper. Cook for 5 minutes until the mushrooms release liquid. Add the snow peas, cabbage, broccoli, kale, and bok choy. Cook for 3 to 4 minutes until the vegetables soften. Add the tofu and sauce, and stir to combine.

4. Serve over cauliflower rice, brown rice, or quinoa, if using, and top with sesame seeds, scallions, and cilantro.

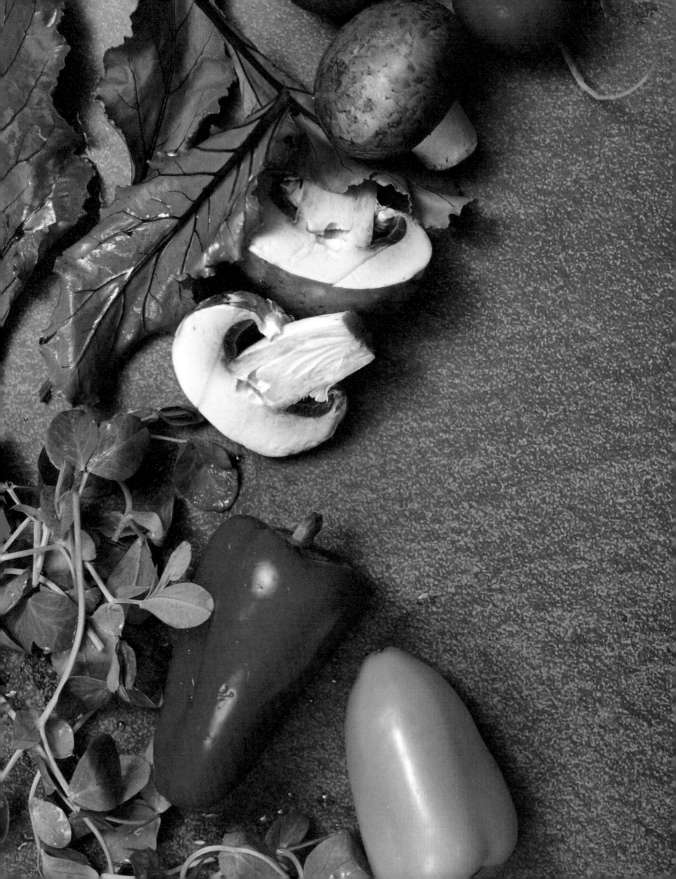

CHAPTER 8
PLATES

Prep Time: 5 minutes
Cook Time: 45–60 minutes
Serves: 4–6

Potato Party

Baked potatoes are the simplest nonrecipe recipe. They are the basis of many other dishes in this book, and they can also be enjoyed plain or with a wide variety of toppings. Make enough to enjoy throughout the week!

4–6 large potatoes of equal size, scrubbed

Topping Suggestions
Salsa
Hummus
Steamed broccoli and
    sesame seeds
Beans and pico de gallo
Chives, dill, and
    unsweetened plain
    vegan yogurt
Marinara sauce and
    fresh basil
Roasted or steamed
    veggies
Nutritional yeast

1. Preheat the oven to 450°F (230°C).

2. Place potatoes directly on the oven rack and bake for 45 to 60 minutes, depending on their size. Add any desired toppings and enjoy immediately, or store in an airtight container in the refrigerator for up to 6 days.

NOTE

Here are six great reasons to incorporate more potatoes into your diet:

- Potatoes have been scientifically determined to be the most satisfying food.[1]

- There are so many types and varieties of potatoes, you can become a connoisseur, and the distinctive flavors become more and more noticeable as your palate shifts.

- Potatoes are ubiquitous. You can find them at any store and order them at most restaurants, where it would be difficult to sneak in butter, oil, or other ingredients without you noticing.

- Potatoes are perfectly portable—you can take them on the road, on an airplane, or anywhere.

- You can store cooked potatoes for several days, so batch cooking them in advance will save you cooking time throughout the week.

- Potatoes are surprisingly nutritious: full of potassium, magnesium, folate, vitamin C, and enough protein that—shockingly—they have a better amino acid profile than lean beef!

Twice-Baked Potatoes
with One-Pan Roasted Veggies

Prep Time: 15 minutes
Cook Time: 1 hour 30 minutes
Serves: 2

These potatoes are part of my regular rotation, and I double or triple the recipe to enjoy throughout the week. They take a bit of time to prepare, but it is mostly hands-off and well worth it for a satisfying, hearty, wholesome dish. Roast whatever veggies you may have in your fridge to turn this into a feel-good, resourceful, tasty, "finish-the-food-in-the-refrigerator" meal.

2 large russet potatoes, scrubbed

1 yellow onion, finely diced

1 cup thinly sliced Brussels sprouts

2 tbsp nutritional yeast

½ cup plant milk, plus more to thin

1 tsp miso paste

1 tsp freshly squeezed lemon juice

¼ cup chopped fresh flat-leaf parsley

Freshly ground black pepper, to taste

2 cups mixed veggies (broccoli florets, asparagus spears, halved Brussels sprouts, and/or cauliflower florets)

1 cup grape or cherry tomatoes

1. Preheat the oven to 450°F (230°C). Place the potatoes directly onto the oven rack, and bake for 60 minutes. Set aside to cool.

2. Heat a large saucepan or Dutch oven over medium-high heat. When hot, sauté the onion with as little water as possible, just enough to avoid burning, for 3 minutes or until translucent. Add the Brussels sprouts, and sauté for 3 to 5 minutes, adding a splash of water as needed to avoid burning, until lightly browned. Remove from the heat, and set aside.

3. When the potatoes have cooled, slice off the tops (lengthwise), and scoop the flesh into a large bowl. Place the scooped-out potato skins on a baking sheet, and set aside.

4. To the bowl with the potato flesh, add the nutritional yeast, plant milk, miso paste, and lemon juice. Mash with a potato masher until well combined. Add the cooked onion and Brussels sprouts mixture, along with the parsley and pepper, and stir to combine. Spoon the mixture into the potato skins. (If the mixture is too stiff to spoon easily, stir in 1 to 2 tablespoons of plant milk to loosen it.)

5. To the baking sheet with the potatoes, add the mixed veggies and tomatoes, spreading them around the potatoes in an even layer. Bake for 20 to 30 minutes until the potatoes are golden brown. Serve immediately.

Chili Cheese Fries

2 large russet potatoes,
cooked and cooled
1 batch **Nacho Squash
Sauce** (page 165)
Sliced scallions,
to garnish

For the chili
1 small red onion, finely
chopped
½ green bell pepper,
finely chopped
1 jalapeño, chopped
small
2 cloves garlic, minced
2 tbsp chili powder
2 tsp ground cumin
1 tsp ground coriander
1 tsp dried Mexican
oregano
1 tsp ancho chili powder
1 tsp smoked paprika
1 (16oz; 450g) pkg
extra-firm tofu,
crumbled
1 (15oz; 425g) can
kidney beans, drained
and rinsed
2 cups crushed
tomatoes
½ cup tomato paste
2 chipotle peppers in
adobo, finely chopped
3 tbsp adobo sauce
1 tbsp reduced-sodium
tamari
1 tsp liquid smoke
1½ cups low-sodium
vegetable broth

Potatoes and chili are a perfect batch-cooking combo!
Baked potatoes are ideal to prepare ahead of time and
enjoy in myriad ways throughout the week, and this
satisfying tofu chili can also be made in advance and
enjoyed over fries or baked potatoes; atop spaghetti
squash, cauliflower rice, or cooked greens; or even as
a salad "dressing" topper. This recipe makes a large
batch of chili; halve it if just using for chili cheese fries.

1. Preheat the oven to 425°F (220°C). Line a baking sheet with
    parchment paper or a silicone baking mat. Cut the precooked
    potatoes into steak fries or rounds, and place them on the prepared
    baking sheet. Set aside.

2. To make the chili, heat a large saucepan or Dutch oven over
    medium-high heat. When hot, sauté the onion with as little water
    as possible, just enough to avoid burning, for 3 minutes or until
    translucent. Add the bell pepper and jalapeño, and cook for 2 to
    3 minutes until the vegetables soften, stirring occasionally. Add the
    garlic, chili powder, cumin, coriander, oregano, ancho chili powder,
    and paprika. Sauté for 60 to 90 seconds, being careful to brown
    but not burn.

3. Add the tofu, kidney beans, crushed tomatoes, tomato paste,
    chipotle peppers, adobo sauce, tamari, liquid smoke, and broth.
    Bring to a boil. When boiling, reduce the heat to low, cover, and
    simmer for 30 minutes or until thick.

4. While the chili simmers, place the fries in the oven, and bake for
    25 to 30 minutes until brown, flipping them midway through.

5. Taste the chili and adjust the seasonings as desired. To serve,
    spoon the chili over the fries, drizzle with Nacho Squash Sauce, and
    sprinkle with scallions. The chili, fries, and sauce can be refrigerated
    in separate airtight containers for up to 5 days.

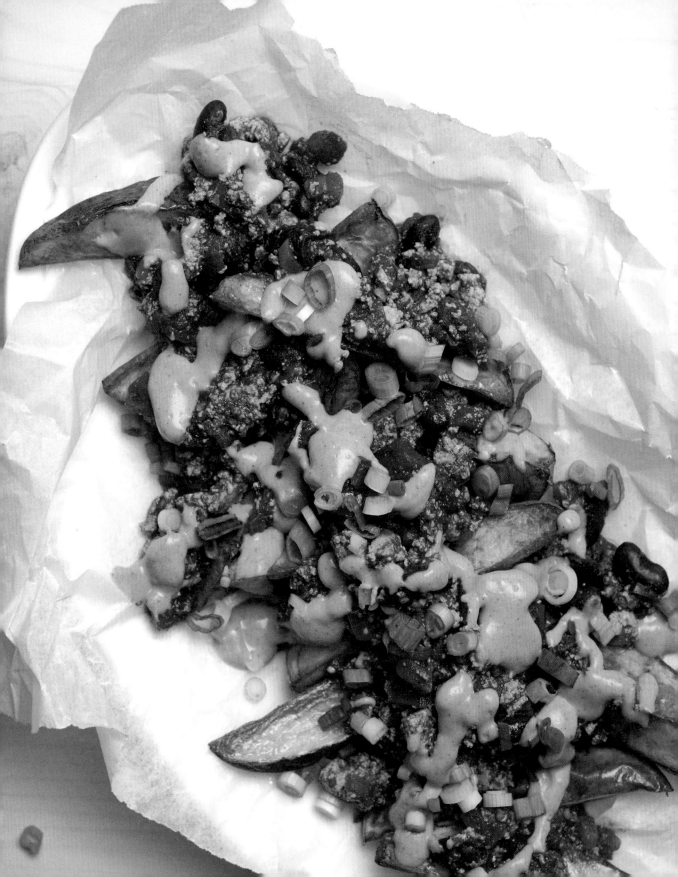

Prep Time: 40 minutes
Cook Time: 60 minutes
Serves: 4–6

Potato–Pea Samosa Patties
with Cilantro–Mint Sauce

Samosas are traditionally a South Asian baked or fried pastry dish with a savory filling. Here, we skip the pastry and turn the filling into spiced potato patties, sprinkled with peas, and topped with a fresh, creamy cilantro-mint sauce. These patties pair deliciously with the Saag Paneer (page 98) for an Indian-inspired meal.

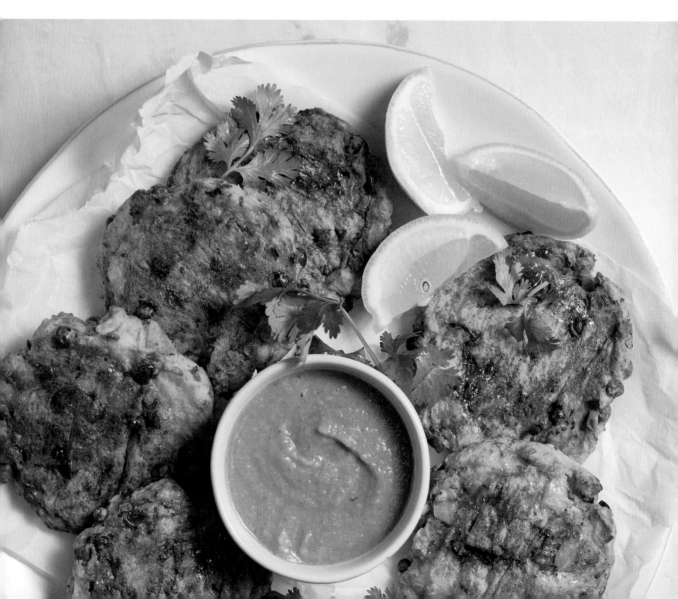

For the patties

3 large russet potatoes, peeled and chopped
¼ tsp cumin seeds
3 cloves garlic, minced
1 tsp ginger paste
2 tbsp finely diced jalapeño
¼ cup plant milk
¾ tsp garam masala
¼ tsp ground turmeric
½ tsp ground coriander
½ tsp ground cumin
1 cup frozen peas, defrosted
1 scallion, finely chopped
1 tbsp freshly squeezed lemon juice
2 tbsp chopped fresh cilantro

For the sauce

1 (15oz; 425g) can Great Northern beans, drained and rinsed
1 cup chopped fresh cilantro
¼ cup chopped fresh mint
2 scallions, chopped
2 tbsp freshly squeezed lemon juice
1 tbsp chopped jalapeño
1 tsp miso paste
½ tsp garlic powder
½ tsp ground cumin
½ cup water

1. To a large saucepan, add the potatoes and enough water to cover by 1 inch (2.5cm). Cover and bring to a boil over high heat. Boil for 15 minutes or until the potatoes are fork-tender. Drain the potatoes, and return them to the pot. Using a potato masher, mash the potatoes. Set aside.

2. Heat a large saucepan over medium-high heat. Toast the cumin seeds until fragrant, about 1 minute. Add the garlic, ginger paste, jalapeño, and 2 tablespoons water. Cook for 30 seconds, stirring. Add the plant milk, garam masala, turmeric, coriander, and cumin along with an additional 1 to 2 tablespoons water as needed to prevent burning. Stir to combine, and remove from heat.

3. Add the mashed potatoes, peas, scallions, lemon juice, and cilantro to the mixture; stir to combine. Allow to cool. (Mixture can be placed in the refrigerator to cool and firm up, and patties can be made the next day if needed.)

4. Meanwhile, to make the sauce, place all sauce ingredients in a high-speed blender and blend until smooth.

5. Preheat the oven to 425°F (220°C), and line a baking sheet with parchment paper or a silicone baking mat. Roll the potato mixture into 2-inch (5cm) balls and place on the prepared baking sheet. Flatten into patties. Bake for 20 minutes, flip the patties, and bake an additional 15 minutes, or until golden brown.

6. Serve warm with the cilantro-mint sauce for dipping. Patties can also be wrapped in a collard green leaf, or served over salad greens with sliced cucumber, red onion, and tomato.

NOTE If you have an air fryer, bake the patties at 400°F (200°C) for 20 minutes.

Prep Time: 10 minutes
Cook Time: 40 minutes
Serves: 2

Christine's Eggplant "Dogs"

This recipe comes from my friend Christine, who has one of those social media feeds that always makes you hungry. Eggplant is one of the top weight loss–friendly foods, as it is filled with fiber without a lot of calories. It is such a versatile veggie, and these "dogs" reflect all of eggplant's potential. Have some fun with these, and experiment with any or all of the fixings. My favorite way to enjoy these so far is with some kimchi and a fork and knife, but I plan on continuing the exploration.

2 medium Japanese eggplants (or 1 medium Italian eggplant, sliced vertically into 4 long wedges)

For the marinade
2 tbsp miso paste
2 tbsp mustard (Chinese hot mustard for zip)
2 tbsp plain vegan yogurt
1 tsp reduced-sodium tamari
1 tsp rice vinegar
2 sprouted-grain hot dog buns or large lettuce leaves, to serve

Optional Toppings
Vegan kimchi
Finely chopped red onion, or sliced green onion
Thinly sliced cucumber
Daikon matchsticks
Thinly sliced avocado
Grated carrot
Thinly sliced jalapeño
Furikake or sesame seeds

1. Preheat the oven to 375°F (190°C). To make the marinade, in a small bowl, whisk together all marinade ingredients until smooth.

2. On a work surface, layer a piece of foil and then a piece of parchment paper large enough to wrap each eggplant (or each wedge). Place the eggplant (or wedge) diagonally on the parchment.

3. Carefully slit each eggplant (or wedge) lengthwise, about three-fourths of the way through. Drizzle the marinade over the slit and the overflow around the eggplant. Tuck the corners of the parchment/foil wraps and roll up the eggplant tightly.

4. Place the eggplant parcels on a baking sheet and roast for 40 minutes. Unwrap, slice off the stems, and serve in a hot dog bun or lettuce wrap with desired toppings.

> NOTE For extra browning, unwrap the eggplant after baking, and place under the broiler for 2 minutes.

Not-So-Crabby Cakes
with Remoulade Sauce

Prep Time: 45 minutes
Cook Time: 30 minutes
Serves: 2–4

Young (unripe) jackfruit comes canned in water or brine and has a texture similar to that of shredded meat. In this recipe, the brine from the jackfruit combined with the nori and Old Bay Seasoning offers a crab-like flavor.

1 (20oz; 567g) can young green jackfruit, drained and rinsed

4 tbsp freshly squeezed lemon juice, divided

¼ sheet nori, shredded

1 cup canned chickpeas

½ cup finely chopped yellow onion

¼ cup finely chopped red bell pepper

1 (15oz; 4525g) can Great Northern beans, drained and rinsed

4 tbsp plant milk

1 tsp low-sodium Old Bay Seasoning

3 tbsp chopped flat-leaf parsley, divided

1 tbsp + ½ tsp yellow mustard, divided

1 tsp freshly ground black pepper, divided

¼ cup roasted red pepper

1 scallion, sliced

1 tbsp ketchup

½ tbsp capers, rinsed

1 tsp anchovy-free Worcestershire sauce

½ tsp hot sauce

¼ tsp garlic powder

Chopped romaine lettuce or salad greens, to serve

1. Preheat the oven to 400°F (200°C), and line a baking sheet with parchment paper or a silicone mat. In a large bowl, mash the jackfruit with a fork to shred. Squeeze out any excess water. Add 3 tablespoons lemon juice and the nori, toss to combine, and set aside.

2. Drain the chickpeas, reserving 1 tablespoon aquafaba (liquid from can). In a food processor, pulse the chickpeas until they resemble breadcrumbs. Add the chickpeas to the jackfruit.

3. Heat a medium saucepan over medium-high heat. When hot, sauté the onion and bell pepper with as little water as possible, just enough to avoid burning, for 5 minutes or until the onion is translucent. Add to the jackfruit mixture.

4. In the food processor, pulse the Great Northern beans, reserved aquafaba, and plant milk until smooth. Add 2 tablespoons of this purée to the jackfruit mixture. Set aside the remaining purée to make the remoulade.

5. To the jackfruit mixture, add the Old Bay Seasoning, 2 tablespoons parsley, ½ teaspoon mustard, and ½ teaspoon pepper; toss to combine. Roll the mixture into small balls, place on the prepared baking sheet, and slightly flatten each ball. Bake for 25 minutes, flipping midway through.

6. Meanwhile, finish the remoulade by adding to the food processor with the reserved purée the remaining 1 tablespoon lemon juice, 1 tablespoon parsley, 1 tablespoon mustard, and ½ teaspoon pepper, as well as the roasted red pepper, scallion, ketchup, capers, Worcestershire, hot sauce, and garlic powder. Blend until smooth.

7. Serve the cakes over a bed of romaine or other salad greens, drizzled with the remoulade sauce.

Prep Time: 20 minutes
Cook Time: 30–35 minutes
Serves: 2

Almond-Crusted Tofu
with Katsu Sauce

Three ingredients found to support hair health and growth are soyfoods, almonds, and capsaicin. This crispy, almond-coated tofu with classic katsu curry sauce is a delicious, nutritious way to enjoy all three in one delicious dish (and maybe boost your hair too!).

¼ cup raw almonds
1 tbsp sesame seeds
1 (16oz; 450g) block
  extra-firm tofu
1 tsp reduced-sodium
  tamari
Raw or steamed greens
  (optional), to serve

For the sauce
½ cup chopped yellow
  onion
1 carrot, chopped
1 clove garlic, minced
½ tbsp minced fresh
  ginger
1 tsp mild curry powder
¼ tsp garam masala
¼ tsp ground turmeric
½ tsp red pepper flakes
½ tbsp tomato paste
½ tbsp arrowroot
  powder
½ cup chopped mango,
  fresh or frozen
1 cup low-sodium
  vegetable broth
1 tbsp reduced-sodium
  tamari
Freshly ground black
  pepper, to taste

1. Preheat the oven to 425°F (220°C). Line a baking sheet with parchment paper or a silicone baking mat.

2. In a blender or food processor, pulse the almonds until coarse like breadcrumbs. Transfer to a small bowl, add the sesame seeds, and toss to combine.

3. Cut the tofu block lengthwise into 4 "steaks". Pat the tofu steaks dry, and then coat them with tamari. Press each tofu steak into the almond sesame mix, coating both sides, and place on the prepared baking sheet. Bake for 20 minutes, flip the tofu steaks, and bake for 10 to 15 minutes more until golden brown.

4. Meanwhile, to make the sauce, heat a medium saucepan or Dutch oven over medium-high heat. When hot, sauté the onion with as little water as possible, just enough to avoid burning, for 3 minutes or until translucent. Add the carrot and 1 tablespoon water (or enough to avoid burning), and cook for 2 to 3 minutes.

5. Add the garlic and ginger, stir, and then add the curry powder, garam masala, turmeric, red pepper flakes, and tomato paste. Stir until fragrant, about 1 minute. Add the arrowroot and 1 tablespoon water, and stir for 30 seconds. Add the mango, broth, and tamari. Stir to combine, and bring to a boil. When boiling, reduce the heat to medium-low, and simmer for 15 minutes or until carrots are soft.

6. Transfer the sauce to a blender, or use an immersion blender in the pot, and purée until smooth. Taste and season with pepper, if needed. To serve, slice the tofu steaks into strips, and plate on a bed of raw or steamed greens, if desired. Drizzle the katsu sauce over the tofu, and enjoy immediately.

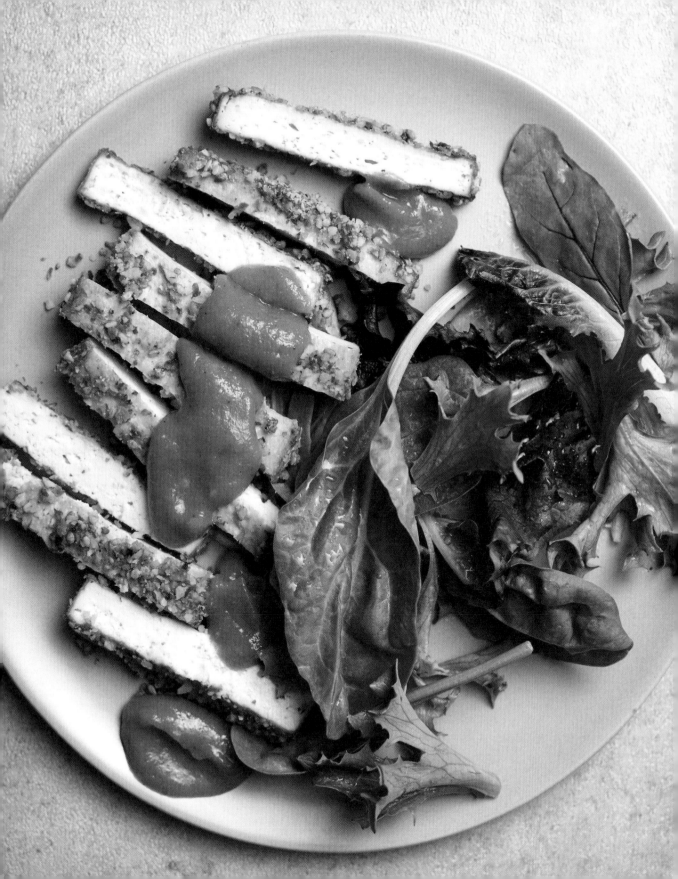

Spicy Peanut-Glazed Eggplant

These spicy, sweet, peanut-buttery flavors pair harmoniously with eggplant's chewy, spongy texture. Enjoy this dish with a side of rice and stir-fried vegetables such as bok choy, broccoli, and cabbage, plus a sprinkle of fresh herbs and sesame seeds.

1 tbsp natural peanut butter

1 tbsp tahini

1 tbsp reduced-sodium tamari

1 tbsp miso paste

2 tsp mirin

1–3 tsp sriracha, to taste

1 tsp minced garlic

½ tsp minced fresh ginger

1 tbsp water

2 medium Japanese eggplants

1. Preheat the oven to 350°F (175°C). Line a baking sheet with parchment paper or a silicone baking mat.

2. In a small bowl, whisk together the peanut butter, tahini, tamari, miso paste, mirin, sriracha, garlic, ginger, and water. Add more water to thin, as needed, to reach a spreadable consistency.

3. Remove the stems of the eggplants, and cut in half lengthwise. Score the cut side in cross hatches deep enough for glaze to penetrate, taking care to not pierce the skin. Place the eggplant on the prepared baking sheet, cut side up, and spread the topping evenly over the flesh. Bake for 20 to 25 minutes until browned, and enjoy immediately.

Crispy Smashed Fingerling Potatoes
with Green Goddess Dressing

Prep Time: 5 minutes
Cook Time: 60 minutes
Serves: 2–4

A twist on standard French fries, smashed potatoes offer more surface area for more crispy goodness. Serve them with the zesty, herbaceous green goddess dressing, or use another dressing, dip, hummus, salsa, or any other way you prefer to potato.

1½ lb (680g) fingerling or baby potatoes
½ tsp garlic powder
½ tsp onion powder
½ tsp paprika
½ tsp freshly ground black pepper

For the dressing
1 cup chopped fresh chives
1 cup chopped fresh cilantro
1 medium jalapeño, deseeded and roughly chopped
2 cloves garlic
4 tbsp tahini
4 tbsp nutritional yeast
2 tbsp miso paste
4 tbsp freshly squeezed lime juice
⅔ cup water
1 tbsp chia seeds

1. To a large saucepan or Dutch oven, add the potatoes and enough water to cover them. Bring to a boil over medium-high heat. When boiling, reduce the heat to medium-low, and simmer for 20 minutes or until fork-tender. Drain the potatoes, and preheat the oven to 450°F (230°C).

2. Line a baking sheet with parchment paper or a silicone baking mat. Place the boiled potatoes on the prepared baking sheet. Using a spatula or the bottom of a mug, smash each potato. Sprinkle the smashed potatoes with the garlic powder, onion powder, paprika, and pepper. Bake for 30 to 35 minutes or until golden brown.

3. To make the dressing, in a blender, purée the chives, cilantro, jalapeño, and garlic for 30 to 60 seconds. Add the tahini, nutritional yeast, miso paste, lime juice, water, and chia seeds. Blend until smooth.

4. Serve the potatoes hot with the dressing as a dip.

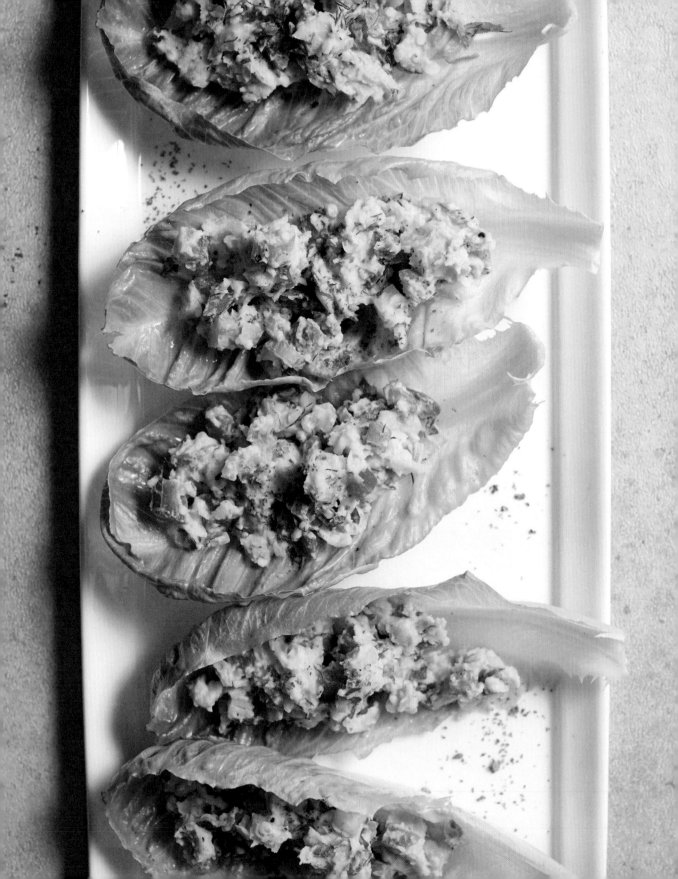

Fresh Butter Bean Smash Lettuce Wraps

Prep Time: 15 minutes
Cook Time: None
Serves: 2

This is a fresh, peppy, and easy everyday salad that my dear friend Sharon shared with me as a staple in her regular rotation. The flavorful beans are delicious in a wrap but can also be served over a big bed of salad greens if you want to dig in with a fork. Za'atar is the perfect topper, adding warmth, and the satisfying crunch of the veggies makes it hard to resist.

1 (15oz; 425g) can butter beans, drained and rinsed
2 celery stalks, finely chopped
3 scallions, thinly sliced
½ red bell pepper (or chile), finely chopped
¼ cup finely chopped fresh flat-leaf parsley
¼ cup dill relish
1 tbsp tahini
1 tbsp chopped fresh dill
½ tbsp freshly squeezed lemon juice
½ tsp freshly ground black pepper or more, to taste
10–12 lettuce leaves, to serve
1 tsp za'atar, to garnish

1. To a large bowl, add the butter beans, and mash until creamy. Add the celery, scallions, bell pepper, parsley, dill relish, tahini, dill, lemon juice, and pepper; stir to combine.

2. To serve, scoop a heaping spoonful of the bean mixture into each lettuce leaf. Sprinkle with za'atar.

Prep Time: 40 minutes
Cook Time: None
Serves: 2

Korean Summer Rolls
with Spicy Peanut Dipping Sauce

Crunchy and fresh, summer rolls are a vibrant and delightful meal to enjoy any time of year. It's fun to mix and match vegetables for added color and creativity. Kimchi gives this version a spicy kick. And who doesn't want another excuse to dip something into a spicy peanut sauce?

6 (9-in; 23cm) rice
  paper wrappers

For the filling
12 romaine lettuce
  leaves, halved
  vertically, ribs
  removed
½ cup chopped kimchi
½ cup shredded carrots
½ cup julienned red bell
  pepper
½ cup julienned
  cucumber
½ cup shredded red
  cabbage
3 scallions, thinly sliced

For the sauce
¼ cup natural peanut
  butter (no added salt,
  sugar, or stabilizers)
2 tbsp rice wine vinegar
2 tbsp freshly squeezed
  lime or lemon juice
2 tsp minced fresh
  ginger
1–2 tbsp sriracha or
  other hot sauce
1 tsp reduced-sodium
  tamari
1 tsp maple syrup
1 tbsp water

1. To make the sauce, in a blender, combine the peanut butter, rice wine vinegar, lime juice, ginger, sriracha, tamari, maple syrup, and water. Blend until smooth, adding more water if needed to thin. Set aside.

2. Gather all filling ingredients on a large plate or in separate bowls. Fill a shallow dish with about 1 inch (2.5cm) of water.

3. Place a wrapper in the water, and soak for 10 to 15 seconds until it softens. Remove and place on a large plate or cutting board lined with a paper towel. Begin adding fillings, starting with the lettuce and then adding a heaping tablespoon each of kimchi, carrot, bell pepper, cucumber, cabbage, and scallion. Carefully fold up the bottom. Fold in the left and right sides, and tuck and roll it over twice, tightly.

4. Repeat to fill the remaining wrappers. Slice each roll in half, and serve immediately with the peanut dipping sauce.

> NOTE You can always substitute sunflower seed butter, cup for cup, for the peanut butter if there is an allergy or preference.

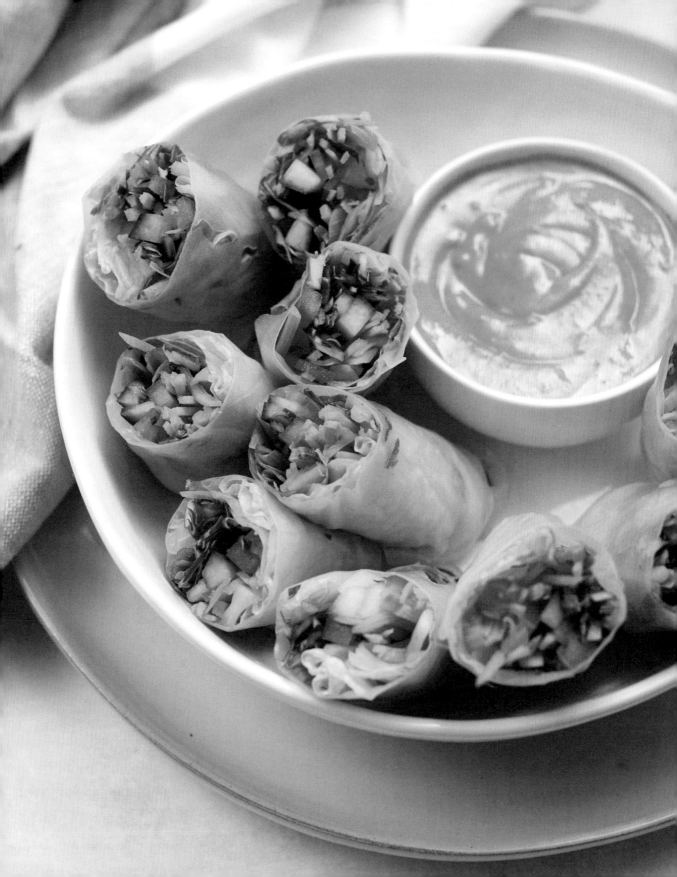

Prep Time: 20 minutes
Cook Time: 10 minutes
Serves: 2

Mushroom Cabbage Cups

Cabbage cups are a delicious way to make eating vegetables fun. This low-calorie, high-nutrition version uses mushrooms as the main star and can be served as a satisfying appetizer or as a side dish.

2 tbsp reduced-sodium tamari
1 tbsp rice vinegar
1 tbsp sweet red chili sauce
1 tsp minced garlic
1 tsp minced fresh ginger
1 tsp arrowroot powder or cornstarch
½–1 tsp red pepper flakes
1 (16oz; 450g) pkg mushrooms, sliced
½ cup chopped red bell pepper
½ cup sliced scallions, plus more to serve
¼ cup chopped celery
¼ cup shredded carrots
1 (8oz; 225g) can water chestnuts, drained, rinsed, and chopped
6–8 cabbage leaves (Savoy, napa, or green; see note)
¼ cup chopped fresh cilantro or Thai basil
Sriracha (optional), to taste

1. In a small bowl, whisk together the tamari, rice vinegar, chili sauce, garlic, ginger, arrowroot, and red pepper flakes.

2. Heat a large saucepan over medium-high heat. When hot, add the mushrooms to the pan, and let them sit until they begin to release liquid. Stir and let some of the liquid reduce, about 5 minutes. Add the bell pepper, scallions, celery, carrots, and water chestnuts. Sauté for 1 to 2 minutes until the vegetables begin to soften. Add the sauce, and stir to combine. Cook for 2 minutes more until the sauce thickens.

3. Spoon the mushroom mixture into the cabbage leaves, and arrange on a serving dish. Sprinkle with cilantro or Thai basil, plus additional scallions and a few drops of sriracha, if using. Enjoy.

NOTE You can substitute lettuce leaves for the cabbage, or plate the filling over shredded cabbage or lettuce, salad-style, if preferred.

Pinto Bean and Corn Jicama Nachos

Prep Time: 20 minutes + preparing sauce
Cook Time: 10 minutes
Serves: 2

Nachos make such a fun meal, as they offer the opportunity to both eat with your hands and pick the perfect bite each time. This version is nutrient-dense and calorie-lean, so you can have all of the fun and pleasure of cheesy, crunchy nachos while still staying on-plan.

1 cup frozen corn kernels

1 (15oz; 425g) can pinto beans, rinsed and drained

2 tsp chili powder

1 tsp chipotle powder

½ tsp smoked paprika

1 tsp freshly squeezed lime juice

1 medium jicama, peeled and sliced into thick disks

½ cup chopped fresh cilantro

¼ cup sliced pickled jalapeños

¼ cup sliced scallions

1 batch **Spicy Cashew Cheesy Sauce** (page 164) or **Nacho Squash Sauce** (page 165)

Hot sauce or salsa, optional

1. In a large saucepan over medium-high heat, heat the corn until it begins to pop and toast, about 5 minutes. Add the beans, chili powder, chipotle powder, and paprika; and smash with a ladle. Cook for 3 minutes or until heated through. Turn off the heat, and drizzle with lime juice.

2. On a serving dish, layer the jicama slices, followed by the bean and corn mixture, cilantro, jalapeños, and scallions. Drizzle the cheesy sauce over top, and add hot sauce or salsa, if desired.

> NOTE Presliced jicama wraps are becoming more widely available, and these make a convenient, time-saving alternative to slicing whole jicama.

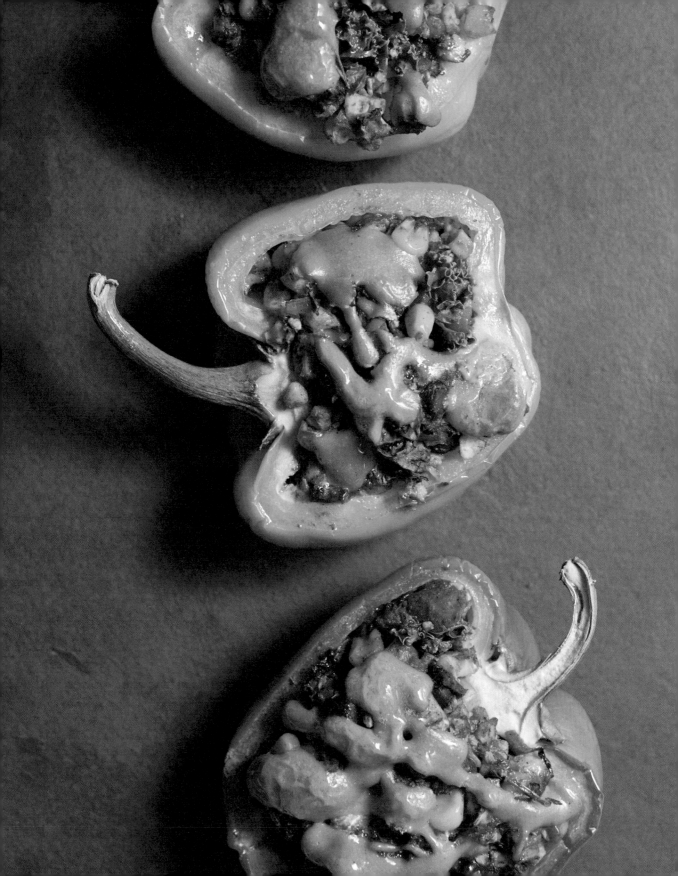

Tex-Mex Stuffed Peppers
with Cheesy Sauce

Prep Time: 10 minutes + preparing sauce
Cook Time: 45 minutes
Serves: 2–4

Comfort food packaged perfectly in peppers. Spicy, creamy nacho cheesy sauce drizzled over hearty, robust cauliflower rice all baked together for a beautiful, satisfying, and delicious treat.

4 large or 5 medium bell peppers (any color)

4 cups cauliflower florets or 1 (16oz; 450g) bag riced cauliflower

1 cup diced yellow onion

3 cloves garlic, minced

¼ cup minced jalapeño

1 cup frozen corn kernels

1 (15oz; 425g) can black beans, drained and rinsed

1 (15oz; 425g) can diced tomatoes

2 tbsp tomato paste

2 tbsp chili powder

1 tsp ground cumin

1 tsp dried oregano

1 tsp smoked paprika

½–1 tsp chipotle powder

2 cups chopped kale

1 cup chopped fresh cilantro

2 tsp freshly squeezed lime juice

1 tsp reduced-sodium tamari

1 tsp liquid smoke (optional)

1 batch **Spicy Cashew Cheesy Sauce** (page 164)

Salsa (optional), to serve

1. Preheat the oven to 350°F (175°C). Line a baking sheet with parchment paper or a silicone baking mat. Slice the peppers in half vertically and remove the seeds. Place the peppers on the baking sheet, cut side up. Bake for 20 minutes until soft but not browned.

2. In a food processor, pulse the cauliflower florets into rice. (This usually needs to be done in batches. Skip this step if using packaged fresh cauliflower rice.)

3. Heat a large saucepan or Dutch oven over medium-high heat. When hot, add the onion and cook with as little water as possible, just enough to avoid burning, for 3 to 4 minutes or until it begins to brown. Add the garlic and cook for 30 to 60 seconds or until the garlic is lightly browned, being careful not to scorch.

4. Add the jalapeño with a splash of water if needed to prevent burning. Cook for 1 to 2 minutes. Add the corn and beans, and stir. Add the cauliflower rice, tomatoes, tomato paste, chili powder, cumin, oregano, paprika, and chipotle powder; stir to combine. Cover, and simmer for 6 to 8 minutes until the cauliflower is cooked through and the sauce is thickened. Add the kale, cover, and simmer for 3 to 4 minutes more until the kale is wilted. Add the cilantro, lime juice, tamari, and liquid smoke, if using. Toss to combine, and remove from the heat.

5. To assemble, fill each roasted pepper halfway with the cauliflower rice mixture, add a few spoonfuls of cheesy sauce, then add more cauliflower rice, and top with cheesy sauce. Place the peppers in a deep casserole dish or Dutch oven, and add ½ cup water to the bottom of the dish. Cover with a lid or foil. Bake for 25 minutes. Serve hot with your favorite salsa, if desired.

Prep Time: 10 minutes
Cook Time: 30–40 minutes
Serves: 2

Grilled Pineapple
with Strawberry Sauce and Black Pepper Balsamic

In this unique play on fruit, the natural sweetness of the pineapple and strawberry is enhanced by grilling and accented with fresh mint, tangy balsamic glaze, and sharp black pepper. Vibrant and well balanced, this colorful plate is a great way to reframe fruit.

1lb (450g) fresh strawberries, stems removed
1 tbsp freshly squeezed lemon juice
1 tsp maple syrup
1 small pineapple, peeled and sliced into wedges
¼ cup finely chopped fresh mint leaves
½ tsp freshly ground black pepper
Balsamic glaze, to garnish

1. In a blender, combine the strawberries and lemon juice, and purée until smooth.

2. Transfer the strawberry mixture to a small saucepan, and bring to a boil over medium-high heat. When boiling, reduce the heat to low, and simmer for 20 to 30 minutes or until reduced by half. Stir in the the maple syrup.

3. Heat a grill pan over medium-high heat. When hot, place the pineapple wedges on the pan, and leave untouched until grill marks appear, about 4 minutes. Flip and repeat on the other side.

4. To serve, drizzle the strawberry sauce over the pineapple. Top with the mint leaves, pepper, and a drizzle of the balsamic glaze. Enjoy immediately.

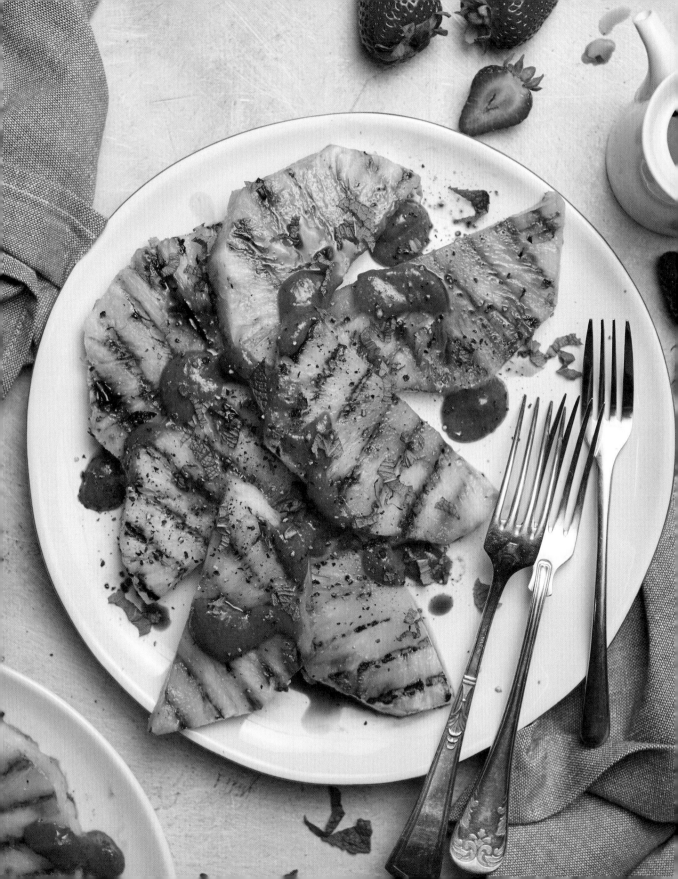

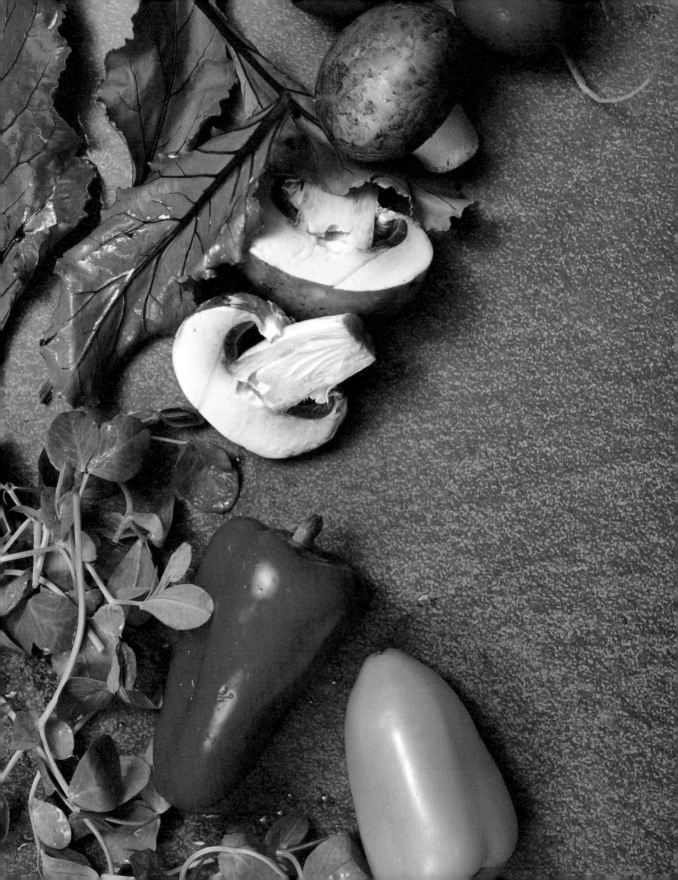

CHAPTER 9

POWER BOWLS

Asian Fusion Salad
with Chickpeas and Balsamic-Tahini Dressing

Prep Time: 20 minutes + 1 hour to marinate
Cook Time: 35 minutes
Serves: 2

Cool, crisp greens and fresh herbs along with warm, sweet-and-spicy roasted chickpeas offer a lovely concert of colors, flavors, and textures. This bowl is reminiscent of Chinese chicken salad—my go-to, all-time favorite salad growing up—but bursting with vibrant, plant-based nutrition.

4 cups garden salad mix or cabbage mix with carrots
4 mandarin oranges, segmented
¼ cup sliced scallions
¼ cup chopped fresh cilantro
1 tsp sesame seeds

For the chickpeas
2 tbsp low-sodium tamari
2 tbsp maple syrup
1 tsp minced fresh ginger
1 tsp minced garlic
½ tsp red pepper flakes
1 (15oz; 425g) can chickpeas, drained, rinsed, and patted dry

For the dressing
2 tbsp balsamic glaze
1 tbsp tahini
½ tsp minced fresh ginger
½ tsp minced garlic
1 tbsp water

1. To make the chickpeas, in a medium food-storage container, whisk together the tamari, maple syrup, ginger, garlic, and red pepper flakes. Add the chickpeas, and toss to combine. Place in the refrigerator, and marinate for at least 1 hour or overnight.

2. Preheat the oven to 425°F (220°C). Line a baking sheet with parchment paper or a silicone baking mat. Drain the marinated chickpeas and spread them on the prepared baking sheet. Roast for 25 to 35 minutes until golden brown, tossing midway.

3. To make the dressing, in a small bowl, whisk together the balsamic glaze, tahini, ginger, garlic, and water until well combined. Add more water to thin, if desired.

4. To assemble, divide the salad mix evenly between 2 serving bowls. To each bowl, add half of the chickpeas and mandarin orange wedges. Drizzle with the dressing; top with the scallions, cilantro, and sesame seeds; and serve immediately.

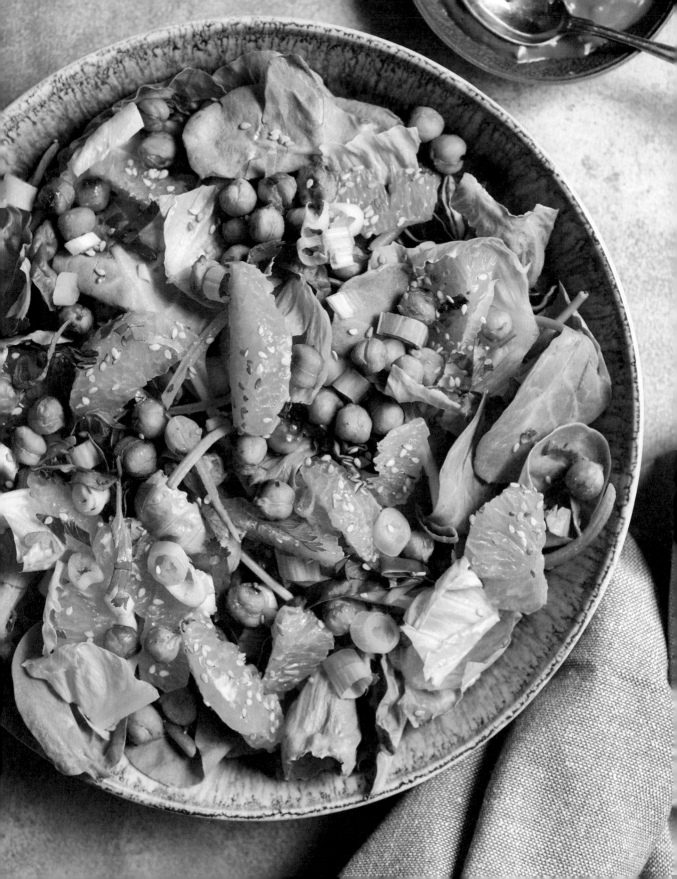

Quick and Easy Burrito Bowl

This toss-it-all-in-one-big-bowl, last-minute, hearty meal is particularly perfect if you have the Mexican Cauliflower Rice prepared ahead of time. If you don't, you can simply swap it out for a package of frozen cauliflower or brown rice, which takes mere minutes to microwave.

1 batch **Mexican Cauliflower Rice** (page 99)
4 cups chopped romaine lettuce
2 cups thinly sliced cabbage (red, green, or a mix)
1 (15oz; 425g) can black or pinto beans, drained and rinsed
1 cup corn kernels (fresh, thawed from frozen, or drained and rinsed from a can)
1 cup halved grape or cherry tomatoes
½ cup finely sliced red onion
½ cup chopped jicama
½ cup salsa
1 medium avocado (optional), sliced thin

To garnish
1 lime, sliced into wedges
½ cup chopped fresh cilantro
Hot sauce, to taste

1. Prepare all of the ingredients. To assemble, fill serving bowls with your desired amount of each item. Drizzle salsa on top, and garnish with lime wedges, cilantro, and hot sauce, to taste.

2. Enjoy immediately, or keep the components (except the avocado) wrapped separately in airtight containers and refrigerate for up to 5 days.

> NOTE This makes for a fun DIY burrito bowl bar you can prepare for loved ones. Kids or others in your home can wrap these ingredients in a warmed tortilla for a burrito or make nachos. For homemade tortilla chips, cut tortillas into wedges, sprinkle them with lime and seasonings as desired, and bake at 400°F (200°C) for 15 to 20 minutes until crispy.

Coleslaw Potato Salad

Prep Time: 10 minutes
Cook Time: 15–20 minutes
Serves: 4–6

It's a picnic in a bowl! We all love coleslaw and potato salad as traditional picnic fare, so why not combine the two with a creamy hemp seed dressing for extra deliciousness? Add pickles, and you have a party.

24oz (680g) petite medley potatoes or fingerling potatoes, quartered
1 (16oz; 450g) bag coleslaw mix
½ cup celery, chopped
¼ cup sliced scallions
¼ cup minced fresh dill
¼ cup minced fresh flat-leaf parsley
1 cup diced dill pickles

For the dressing
1 cup hemp seeds
3 cloves garlic, minced
2 tbsp apple cider vinegar
3 tbsp nutritional yeast
2 tbsp stone-ground mustard (or yellow or Dijon)
1 tbsp maple syrup or molasses
1 tbsp reduced-sodium tamari
1 tsp celery seed
¼ tsp freshly ground black pepper
½ cup water (or more according to preferred thickness)

1. To a large saucepan, add the potatoes and enough water to cover by 2 inches (5cm). Bring to a boil over medium-high heat. Reduce the heat to low, and simmer for 15 to 20 minutes until the potatoes can be pierced easily with a fork. Drain the potatoes, and set aside.

2. To make the dressing, in a blender, combine all dressing ingredients and blend for 60 to 90 seconds until smooth.

3. In a large serving bowl, combine the potatoes, coleslaw mix, celery, scallions, dill, parsley, and pickles. Pour the dressing over the mixture, and toss to combine. Serve immediately, or refrigerate to allow flavors to marinate, and serve cold.

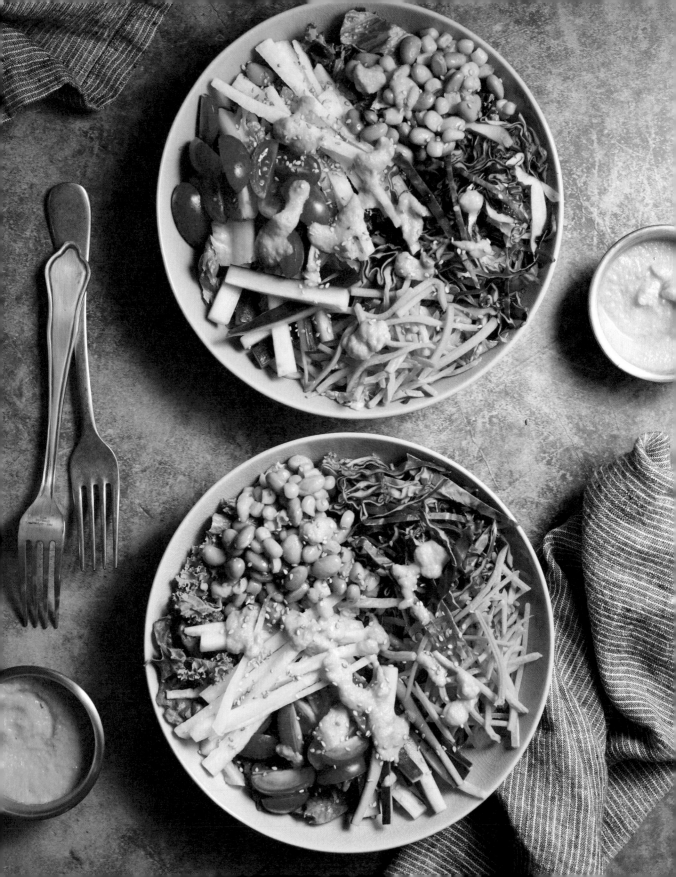

Japanese Rainbow Salad
with Carrot-Ginger Dressing

Prep Time: 20 minutes
Cook Time: 10 minutes
Serves: 2

One of my favorite menu items at Japanese restaurants has always been the simple green salad with the amazing carrot-ginger dressing. That sweet and spicy dressing transformed a plain, boring side salad into something special. This meal-sized version includes edamame, corn, red cabbage, and tomatoes to make a light, colorful, and vibrant bowl.

For the dressing
2 cups sliced carrot
1 celery stalk, chopped
¼ cup chopped apple
¼ cup peeled and
   chopped orange
1 small shallot, chopped
1 tbsp tahini
1 tbsp minced fresh
   ginger
1 tbsp reduced-sodium
   tamari
½ tbsp miso paste
¼ cup rice wine vinegar
¼ cup plant milk
½ tsp freshly ground
   black pepper, or more
   to taste

**For the wasabi
   edamame**
1 cup frozen edamame
1 cup frozen corn
2 tsp reduced-sodium
   tamari
½–1 tsp wasabi powder
½ tsp sesame seeds,
   plus more to garnish

For the salad
2 cups chopped
   romaine lettuce or
   other salad greens
1 small daikon radish,
   peeled and julienned
1 cup shredded red
   cabbage
½ cup julienned carrot
½ cup julienned
   cucumber
½ cup quartered grape
   tomatoes
Sesame seeds
   (optional), to serve

1. To make the dressing, in a high-speed blender, combine all dressing ingredients. Blend until smooth, and set aside.

2. To make the wasabi edamame, to a small bowl, add the edamame, corn, tamari, wasabi powder, and sesame seeds. Toss to combine.

3. Place a medium saucepan over medium-high heat. Add the edamame and corn mixture, and cook until golden brown, adding 1 tablespoon water if necessary, and stirring to avoid burning. Remove from the heat, and set aside.

4. To assemble, divide the lettuce, radish, cabbage, carrots, cucumber, and tomatoes evenly between 2 bowls. Top each bowl with wasabi edamame and drizzle with dressing. Garnish with additional sesame seeds, if desired, and enjoy immediately. Store additional dressing in an airtight container in the refrigerator for up to 4 days.

Immunity Bowl

Eating a whole food, plant-based diet supports a healthy microbiome, which is a primary defender of your health. This bowl highlights some of the top immune-boosting foods—cauliflower, which contains almost three-quarters of the daily recommended intake of vitamin C; mushrooms, which are loaded with immunoprotective compounds; cruciferous veggies and leafy greens, full of sulfur-containing compounds and phytonutrients; garlic, which is anti-inflammatory and antimicrobial; and sauerkraut, with its beneficial probiotics.

1 small head cauliflower, florets separated
2 tsp za'atar
1 tbsp nutritional yeast (optional)
3 tsp reduced-sodium tamari, divided
8oz (225g) shiitake or cremini mushrooms, sliced
2 cloves garlic, minced
1 tbsp minced fresh thyme (or 1 tsp dried)
½ tsp freshly ground black pepper
2 cups packed baby kale or baby spinach, chopped
4 cups mixed salad greens, ideally with cruciferous vegetables
1 (15oz; 425g) can Great Northern beans, drained and rinsed
½ cup sauerkraut

For the dressing
2 tbsp tahini
2 tbsp freshly squeezed lemon juice
2 cloves garlic
1 tbsp za'atar
1 tbsp reduced-sodium tamari
½ cup water

To garnish (optional)
Sliced scallions
Sesame seeds
Hot sauce

1. Preheat the oven to 425°F (220°C). Line a baking sheet with parchment paper or a silicone baking mat.

2. In a medium bowl, toss the cauliflower with the za'atar, nutritional yeast (if using), and 1 teaspoon tamari. Spread the cauliflower on the prepared baking sheet, and roast for 20 to 25 minutes until tender and the edges are golden brown.

3. Meanwhile, heat a medium saucepan over medium-high heat. Add the mushrooms, garlic, and thyme, along with a few tablespoons of water. Cover, and allow the mushrooms to release their liquid. Remove the cover, and continue cooking until the liquid cooks off, about 5 minutes. Add the remaining 2 teaspoons tamari, pepper, and kale and allow to wilt, stirring frequently. Remove from the heat and set aside.

4. To make the dressing, in a blender, combine all dressing ingredients. Blend until smooth.

5. To assemble, divide the salad greens evenly between 2 serving bowls. To each bowl, add an equal portion of beans, sauerkraut, roasted cauliflower, mushroom mixture, and dressing. Garnish with sliced scallions, sesame seeds, and hot sauce, as desired.

Cuban-Inspired Cilantro-Lime Bowl

Prep Time: 20 minutes
Cook Time: 30 minutes
Serves: 2–4

A much underappreciated starchy fruit—plantains—round out the Cuban-inspired ingredients in this substantial and satisfying bowl. With a thick and creamy bean-based dressing and cauliflower rice standing in for the traditional white rice, this bowl is lightened up, filled with fiber and phytonutrients, and perfectly on plan.

2 large ripe plantains, peeled and cut into ½-in (1.25cm) rounds
¼–1 tsp red pepper flakes, to taste
4 cups coleslaw mix

For the dressing
1 (15oz; 425g) can low-sodium cannellini beans, drained and rinsed
½ cup chopped fresh cilantro
¼ cup nutritional yeast
2 tbsp tahini
2 tbsp reduced-sodium tamari
2 tbsp freshly squeezed lime juice
1 tbsp maple syrup
⅛ tsp red pepper flakes
½ cup plant milk

For the cauliflower rice
1 small yellow onion, chopped
1 (16oz; 450g) pkg cauliflower rice
1 (15oz; 425g) can black beans, drained and rinsed
6 tbsp freshly squeezed lime juice
1 cup chopped fresh cilantro
1 tbsp reduced-sodium tamari

1. Preheat the oven to 400°F (200°C). Line a baking sheet with parchment paper or a silicone baking mat. Place the plantain rounds on the prepared baking sheet, and sprinkle with red pepper flakes. Bake for 10 minutes, flip, and bake for 10 minutes more. Set aside.

2. To make the dressing, in a small blender, combine all ingredients, and blend until smooth. Set aside.

3. To make the cauliflower rice, heat a large saucepan or Dutch oven over medium-high heat. When hot, sauté the onion with as little water as possible, just enough to avoid burning, until it is translucent, about 3 minutes. Add the cauliflower rice and ¼ cup water. Stir and sauté until the vegetables soften. Add the black beans, and cook until warmed. Add the lime juice, cilantro, and tamari, and stir to combine. Remove from the heat.

4. To assemble, plate the cauliflower rice, coleslaw mix, and plantains, and drizzle with dressing. Serve immediately.

Prep Time: 5 minutes +
1 hour to marinate +
preparing croutons and
dressing
Cook Time: 30 minutes
Serves: 2

Tempeh Reuben Salad
with Rye Potato Croutons and Russian Dressing

Is there anything more decadent and delicious than a tempeh Reuben? In my humble opinion, I can't think of anything more irresistible. So, then, make it as healthy as possible, and still enjoy the salty, sour sauerkraut and the hearty, starchy rye along with a sweet Russian dressing for the full effect and amped-up nutrition. The rye potato croutons are worth the extra effort as they are the best thing since sliced bread!

4 tbsp reduced-sodium tamari

2 tbsp maple syrup

2 tbsp apple cider vinegar

1 tsp liquid smoke

½ tsp smoked paprika

1 (8oz; 225g) pkg tempeh, cut into small, even pieces

4 cups garden salad blend (or a mix of iceberg or romaine lettuce, cabbage, and carrots)

½ cup sauerkraut

½ cup grape tomatoes, sliced

1 batch **Rye Potato Croutons** (page 92)

1 batch **Russian Dressing** (page 153)

1. To a medium storage container, add the tamari, maple syrup, apple cider vinegar, liquid smoke, and paprika. Stir to combine, add the tempeh, and toss. Cover, and marinate in the refrigerator for at least 1 hour or overnight.

2. Preheat the oven to 350°F (175°C). Line a baking sheet with parchment paper or a silicone baking mat. Arrange the tempeh in a single layer on the prepared baking sheet. Bake for 15 minutes, turn over, and bake for 15 minutes more.

3. To assemble, divide the salad greens, sauerkraut, tomatoes, and tempeh evenly between 2 salad bowls. Drizzle with dressing and sprinkle with croutons. Enjoy immediately.

> **NOTE** This salad takes time to prep, but it is well worth it! If you love a Reuben sandwich the way I always have, it is a must-try. You can prep the tempeh, croutons, and dressing ahead of time to expedite the process.

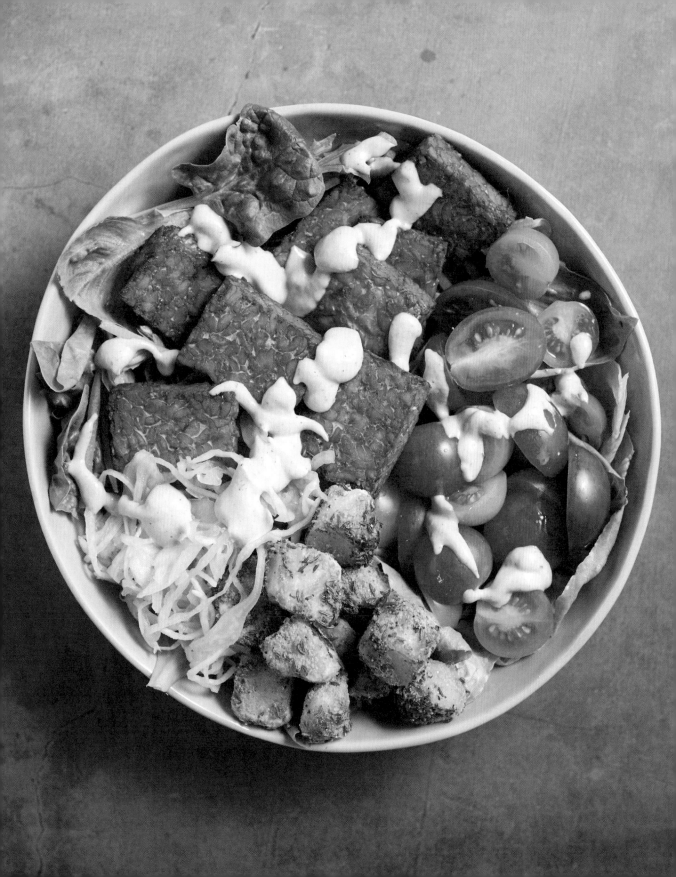

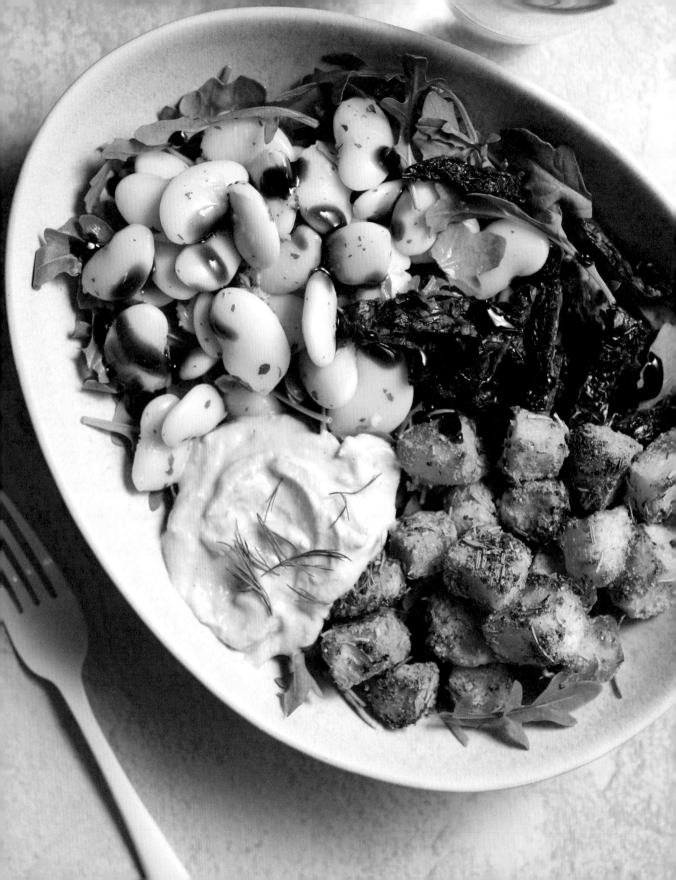

Athena Greek Salad Bowl
with Almond Tzatziki Whip

Prep Time: 30 minutes + 30 minutes to marinate + preparing croutons
Cook Time: 1 minute
Serves: 2

Athena, the ancient Greek goddess associated with wisdom and war, represents this salad bowl because of its strengthening ingredients and Mediterranean flair. With a rainbow of color and a variety of textures, this fresh, unique power bowl gives new meaning to protectress.

1 (15oz; 425g) can butter beans, drained and rinsed
1 tbsp red wine vinegar
1 tbsp freshly squeezed lemon juice
1 tsp dried parsley
4 cups salad greens, such as arugula
½ cup sliced sun-dried tomatoes (not packed in oil)
1 batch **Cheesy Rosemary Potato Croutons** (page 92)
Balsamic glaze, to garnish

For the tzatziki whip
½ cup raw almonds
½ English cucumber, peeled and shredded, divided
3 cloves garlic, sliced
2 tbsp chopped fresh dill
1 tbsp freshly squeezed lemon juice
1 tbsp apple cider vinegar
1 tbsp reduced-sodium tamari
¼ tsp freshly ground black pepper

1. To a medium storage container, add the butter beans, red wine vinegar, lemon juice, and parsley; toss to fully coat the beans. Cover, and place in the refrigerator to marinate for at least 30 minutes or overnight.

2. Prepare the tzatziki whip. In a small saucepan, bring 2 cups water to a boil. Add the almonds, and boil for 1 minute. Drain the almonds and shock with cold water. Using your fingers, gently squeeze the almonds to remove the skins. Discard the skins. In a high-speed blender, combine the blanched almonds, half of the cucumber, garlic, dill, lemon juice, apple cider vinegar, tamari, and pepper. Blend until smooth. Add the remaining cucumber, and pulse once or twice to combine, leaving a bit of chunky texture.

3. Divide the salad greens evenly between 2 salad bowls. Top each bowl with the sun-dried tomatoes, marinated butter beans, potato croutons, and tzatziki whip. Drizzle with the balsamic glaze, and serve immediately.

> NOTE This salad is best made fresh. If making ahead, store all components separately in the refrigerator and assemble just before eating. Reheat or roast the potatoes immediately prior to serving for the best result.

Prep Time: 15 minutes
Cook Time: 35 minutes
Serves: 2–3

Roasted Eggplant Salad

I fell in love with the idea of a "hot and cold" salad after enjoying many iterations while visiting the Middle East many years ago. Combining temperatures, flavors, and textures takes a salad to the next level . . . and I am passionate about next-level salad! This makes for yet another joyful way to serve leftovers and endless opportunities to create deliciousness.

1 large eggplant, cubed
½ yellow onion, diced
1 red bell pepper, diced
6 cloves garlic
1 cup crushed tomatoes
½ cup water
1–3 tsp red pepper flakes, to taste
1 tbsp ground turmeric
1 tsp ground cumin
¼ cup chopped fresh flat-leaf parsley
2 tsp freshly squeezed lemon juice
1 tsp maple syrup
Salad greens or arugula, to serve

1. Preheat the oven to 400°F (200°C). Line a baking sheet with parchment paper or a silicone baking mat. Spread the eggplant, onion, and bell pepper on the prepared baking sheet.

2. Fold each garlic clove into parchment paper, wrap them in foil, and then place the packets on the baking sheet with the vegetables. Bake for 30 minutes or until the vegetables are browned. Remove the baking sheet from the oven, and unwrap the garlic cloves. Chop the roasted garlic.

3. Heat a saucepan or Dutch oven over medium-high heat. When hot, add the roasted vegetables, roasted garlic, crushed tomatoes, water, red pepper flakes, turmeric, and cumin. Sauté, stirring frequently, for 5 minutes or until all the liquid has been absorbed. Stir in the parsley, lemon juice, and maple syrup; remove from the heat. Serve immediately over a bed of salad greens or arugula.

Polenta
with Red Wine Glazed Mushrooms

Prep Time: 15 minutes
Cook Time: 15–20 minutes
Serves: 2

So much romance in one bowl! Hearty polenta and glazed mushrooms with red wine undertones interact in perfect harmony for a beautifully colorful, elegant, and sexy meal that feels like a date night.

3 cups water
1 cup instant polenta
2 tbsp nutritional yeast
1 tbsp cornstarch
1 cup low-sodium
   vegetable broth,
   divided
1 shallot, minced
4 cloves garlic, minced
16oz (450g) shiitake or
   cremini mushrooms,
   sliced
1 tbsp minced fresh
   rosemary (or 1 tsp
   dried rosemary)
1 tbsp minced fresh
   flat-leaf parsley (or
   1 tsp dried parsley),
   plus more to serve
1 tbsp minced thyme (or
   1 tsp dried thyme)
2 tsp reduced-sodium
   tamari
½ tsp freshly ground
   black pepper
½ cup red wine (or
   ¼ cup balsamic
   vinegar)
5oz (140g) baby
   spinach or kale,
   roughly chopped
2 tbsp balsamic glaze

1. In a small saucepan, bring the water to a boil over medium-high heat. Gradually stir in the polenta, and reduce the heat to medium-low. Cook for about 5 minutes, stirring occasionally. Remove from the heat, cover, and let stand for 2 to 3 minutes. Stir in the nutritional yeast, and set aside.

2. In a small bowl, whisk together the cornstarch and 1 tablespoon broth to create a slurry. Set aside.

3. Heat a large sauté pan over medium-high heat. When hot, add the shallot and 1 tablespoon broth, and cook for 3 minutes until beginning to brown. Add the garlic and 1 tablespoon broth. Sauté for 30 to 60 seconds.

4. Add the mushrooms, rosemary, parsley, thyme, and 2 tablespoons broth. Cover, and let the mushrooms sweat for 2 to 3 minutes until their liquid is released. Remove the lid, and let the liquid dissipate. Add the remaining broth 1 tablespoon at a time, allowing the liquid to evaporate between each addition, until the mushrooms are browned. When the liquid is gone, add the tamari and pepper. Add the slurry, and cook 3 to 5 minutes until the sauce has thickened and reduced. Add the spinach, cover, and turn off the heat to wilt the spinach. Stir and remove from the heat.

5. Divide the polenta evenly between 2 serving bowls, and top each serving with the mushroom mixture. Garnish with balsamic glaze and additional fresh parsley, as desired.

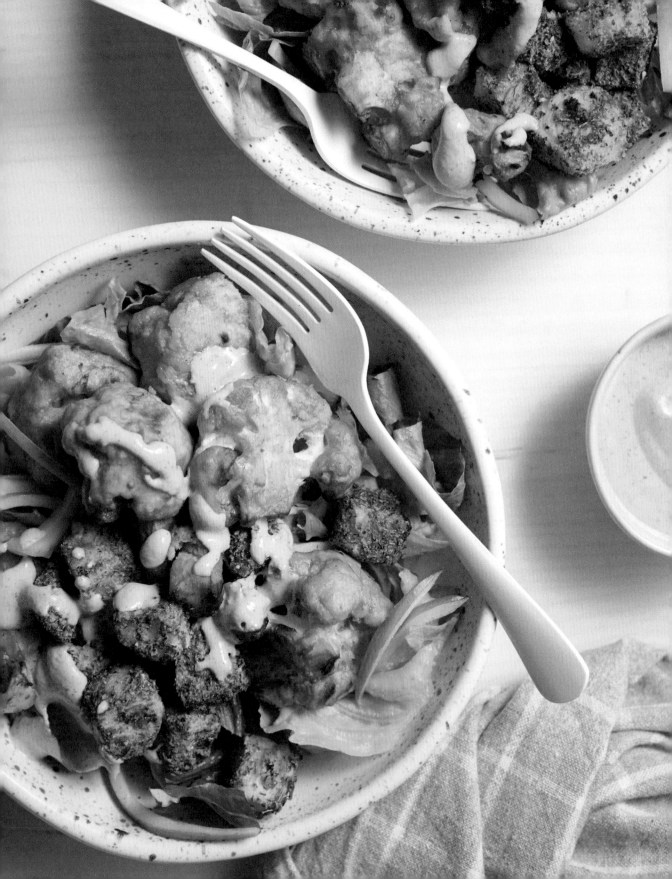

Buffalo Cauliflower Salad
with Hemp Seed Ranch Dressing

Prep Time: 25 minutes + preparing croutons
Cook Time: 35 minutes
Serves: 2–4

This is a popular "plantified" dish that appears on the menu at many plant-based restaurants, but the execution is usually fried, greasy, and lacking in freshness. Well, here is that healthful version—perfectly crisp and clean but feeling like decadence! Enjoy this wholeheartedly, knowing that nutritious absolutely can taste delicious, and stay straight on your plan, too.

½ cup chickpea flour
½ cup water
1 head cauliflower, chopped into large florets
¼ cup lower-sodium buffalo sauce or other hot sauce
4 cups chopped romaine lettuce
1 cup chopped celery
¼ cup thinly sliced red onion
1 batch **Ranch Potato Croutons** (page 92)

For the dressing
½ cup hemp seeds
2 tbsp nutritional yeast
2 tbsp chopped fresh dill
2 tbsp chopped fresh chives
1 tbsp chopped fresh flat-leaf parsley
2½ tsp apple cider vinegar
1½ tsp freshly squeezed lemon juice
1 tsp anchovy-free Worcestershire sauce
1 tsp onion powder
1 tsp garlic powder
¼ tsp freshly ground black pepper
½ cup plant milk

1. Preheat oven to 450°F (230°C). Line a baking sheet with parchment paper or a silicone baking mat.

2. In a large bowl, whisk the chickpea flour with the water until smooth. Place the cauliflower florets in the batter, and turn with a large spoon until lightly coated. Arrange on the prepared baking sheet, and bake for 15 minutes. Flip over and bake 10 minutes more. Remove from the oven, and place in a large bowl. Add the buffalo sauce, and toss to coat. Return to the baking sheet, and bake for 10 minutes more. Set aside.

3. To make the dressing, in a high-speed blender, combine all dressing ingredients and blend until smooth.

4. To serve, plate the lettuce, celery, and onion in large bowls. Toss to combine. Place the cauliflower and potato croutons on top, and drizzle with dressing.

Prep Time: 30 minutes
Cook Time: 30 minutes
Serves: 2

Harissa-Roasted Kabocha Salad Bowl

Kabocha—also called Japanese pumpkin—is a winter squash that has a unique, velvety texture and slightly sweet, rich flavor. Here, this nutritious, carotenoid-rich squash is combined with wholesome quinoa, tomatoes, and greens and flavored with ingredients from the Middle East—spicy harissa and a za'atar-spiced lemon tahini dressing.

1 kabocha squash, sliced into thin wedges
2 tbsp harissa paste
1 cup cherry or grape tomatoes
1 cup quinoa, rinsed
1½ cups water
4 cups kale slaw or salad blend (or substitute 3 cups thinly sliced kale and 1 cup thinly sliced cabbage)
4 medium roasted beets (optional), chopped

For the dressing
2 tbsp tahini
1 tbsp freshly squeezed lemon juice
1 tsp za'atar
1–2 tsp warm water to thin, as desired

1. Preheat the oven to 400°F (200°C). Line a baking sheet with parchment paper or a silicone baking mat.

2. Brush the kabocha wedges with harissa paste, place on the prepared baking sheet, and bake for 15 minutes. Flip the wedges, add the tomatoes to the pan, and bake for 10 to 15 minutes more until the squash is beginning to brown.

3. To a small saucepan, add the quinoa, and toast over medium heat until the quinoa is dry from the rinse and begins to toast. Add the water, and bring to a boil. When boiling, reduce the heat to low, cover, and simmer for 10 to 15 minutes or until all the water is absorbed. Remove from the heat, keep covered, and allow to steam for 5 minutes. Fluff with a fork and set aside.

4. To make the dressing, in a jar or deep cup, combine the tahini, lemon juice, and za'atar. Stir until the mixture is well combined and begins to thicken. Add the warm water, 1 teaspoon at a time, stir, and continue until desired thinness is achieved.

5. To assemble, divide the kale slaw and quinoa evenly between 2 serving bowls. To each bowl, add kabocha wedges, tomatoes, and beets, if using. Top with dressing, and enjoy immediately.

Berry Quinoa Salad

Prep Time: 10 minutes
Cook Time: 25 minutes
Serves: 2

Sweeten up your salad with fresh berries and toasted quinoa. A rainbow of color, flavor, and texture in a bowl, this is a delicious summer dish that is simple and elegant.

1 cup quinoa, rinsed
1 ½ cups water
4 cups baby spinach
½ cup thinly sliced red onion
1 cup blueberries
1 cup sliced strawberries
1 cup raspberries
1 cup blackberries

For the dressing
4 tbsp balsamic glaze
2 tbsp tahini
1 tsp minced fresh ginger
1 tsp minced garlic
3–4 tbsp warm water to thin, as desired

1. To a small saucepan, add the quinoa, and toast over medium heat until the quinoa is dry from the rinse and begins to toast. Add the water, and bring to a boil. When boiling, reduce the heat to low, cover, and simmer for 10 to 15 minutes until all the water is absorbed. When the water is absorbed, remove from the heat, keep covered, and allow the quinoa to steam for 10 minutes. Fluff with a fork, and set aside.

2. To make the dressing, in a medium bowl, whisk together all dressing ingredients until well combined.

3. To assemble, divide the spinach, onion, and quinoa evenly between 2 serving bowls. To each bowl, add an equal amount of berries. Drizzle with dressing, and enjoy immediately.

NOTE Berries can be mixed, according to availability and preference.

Forbidden Sushi Bowl

Sushi in a bowl offers all of the balanced flavors, textures, and colors of sushi plus—added bonus—you can make different combinations for each bite with your fork! Forbidden black rice is a medium-grain heirloom rice that has a deep purple hue and a nutty, slightly sweet flavor. It is rich in anthocyanins, which are phytonutrient pigments that give the rice its unique color.

2 tbsp maple syrup
1 tsp minced
   fresh ginger
1 tsp minced garlic
2 tbsp + 1 tsp reduced-
   sodium tamari, divided
1 (16oz; 450g) pkg
   extra-firm tofu,
   pressed, if desired,
   and cut into 1-in
   (2.5cm) cubes
2 tsp rice vinegar
1 tsp wasabi powder
2 cups cooked
   forbidden black rice
1 cup julienned red
   bell pepper
1 cup julienned
   cucumber
1 cup julienned carrot
1 cup pea shoots
½ avocado, sliced
2 nori sheets, cut into
   strips
2 tsp sliced scallions
1 tsp sesame seeds
   (optional)

1. To a medium storage container, add the maple syrup, ginger, garlic, and 2 tablespoons tamari. Stir to combine. Add the tofu, and toss to coat. Cover, place in the refrigerator, and marinate for at least 1 hour or overnight.

2. Preheat the oven to 400°F (200°C). Line a baking sheet with parchment paper or a silicone baking mat. Place the marinated tofu on the prepared baking sheet. Bake for 20 to 30 minutes until browned, flipping the tofu midway through cooking.

3. In a small bowl, whisk together the rice vinegar, wasabi powder, remaining 1 teaspoon tamari.

4. To assemble, divide the rice, tofu, bell pepper, cucumber, carrot, pea shoots, avocado, nori, and scallions evenly between 2 bowls. Drizzle a bit of the rice vinegar-tamari mixture over each bowl. Sprinkle with the sesame seeds, if using.

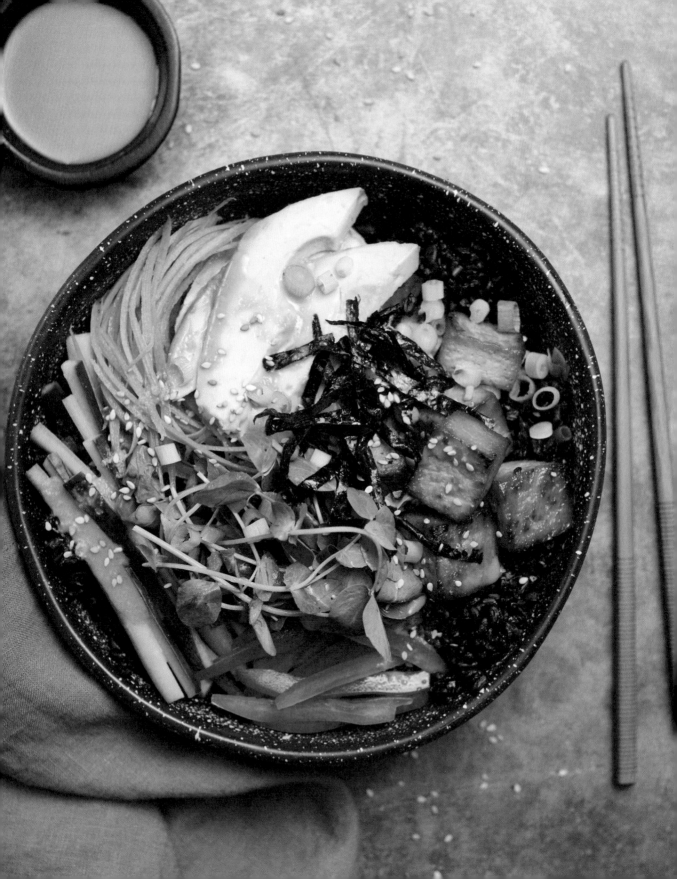

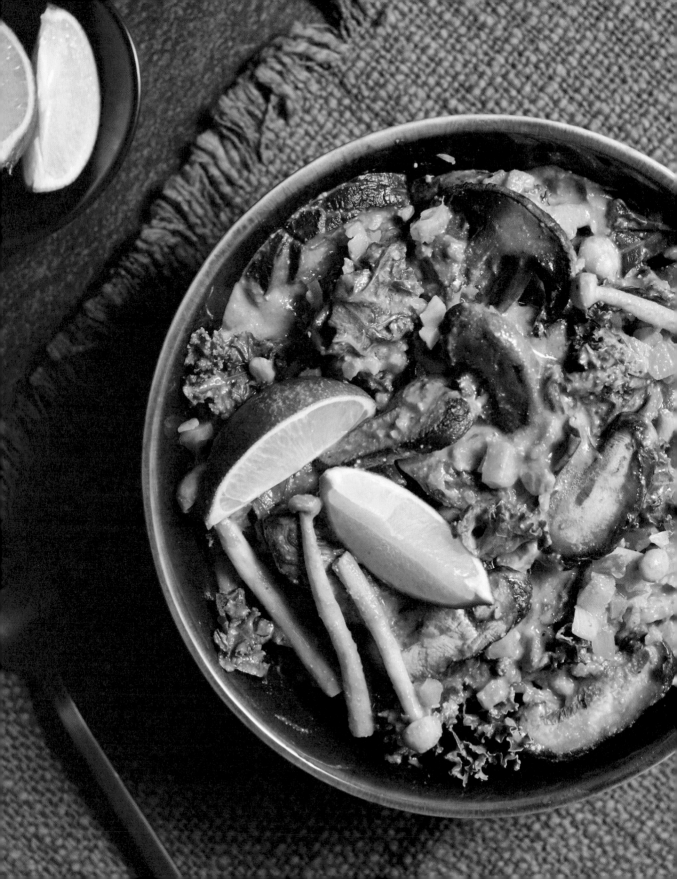

Sriracha Mushroom Cauliflower Rice Bowl

Prep Time: 20 minutes
Cook Time: 25 minutes
Serves: 2–3

Mushrooms are nutritious, offer a toothsome mouthfeel with very few calories, and absorb flavor magnificently, so I wanted to pack as many as possible into this dish. It's a satiating bowl of healthfulness that is infused with a creamy, spicy cashew-based sauce.

4 cups cauliflower florets or 1 (16oz; 450g) pkg cauliflower rice

½ cup raw cashews

3 tbsp nutritional yeast

1 cup roasted red bell peppers (jarred in water)

2 cloves garlic, minced

3 tbsp sriracha

2 tbsp freshly squeezed lemon juice

1 tbsp arrowroot powder

20oz (565g) mixed fresh mushrooms, roughly chopped

5–6 tbsp low-sodium vegetable broth, divided

1 yellow onion, diced

1 tsp reduced-sodium tamari

5oz (140g) mixed greens, roughly chopped

1. In a food processor, pulse the cauliflower florets into rice. You may need to work in batches, depending on the container size. (Skip this step if using prericed cauliflower.)

2. In a high-speed blender, combine the cashews, nutritional yeast, roasted red peppers, garlic, sriracha, lemon juice, and arrowroot. Purée for 60 to 90 seconds until smooth and well combined.

3. Heat a large sauté pan over medium-high heat. Sauté the mushrooms in batches, adding just enough mushrooms in each batch to cover the surface of the pan—don't crowd them too much. Add 1 tablespoon broth per batch. Cook for 3 to 5 minutes until browned, stirring just enough to keep them from sticking. When browned, push the mushrooms to the side, and add another batch of mushrooms and a little more broth. Repeat until all of the mushrooms have been sautéed and are together in the pan. Add the onion with the last batch of mushrooms. There will be a significant amount of fond on the pan, and the mushrooms will be browned and sizzling. Add the tamari and 2 tablespoons broth to deglaze the pan, scraping up the browned bits stuck to the bottom.

4. Add the cauliflower rice and blended sauce, and stir to combine. Reduce the heat, and cook for 10 to 15 minutes until thickened, stirring frequently. Add the greens, turn off the heat, and stir until the greens are wilted. Enjoy immediately, or cool to room temperature, and refrigerate in an airtight container for up 5 days.

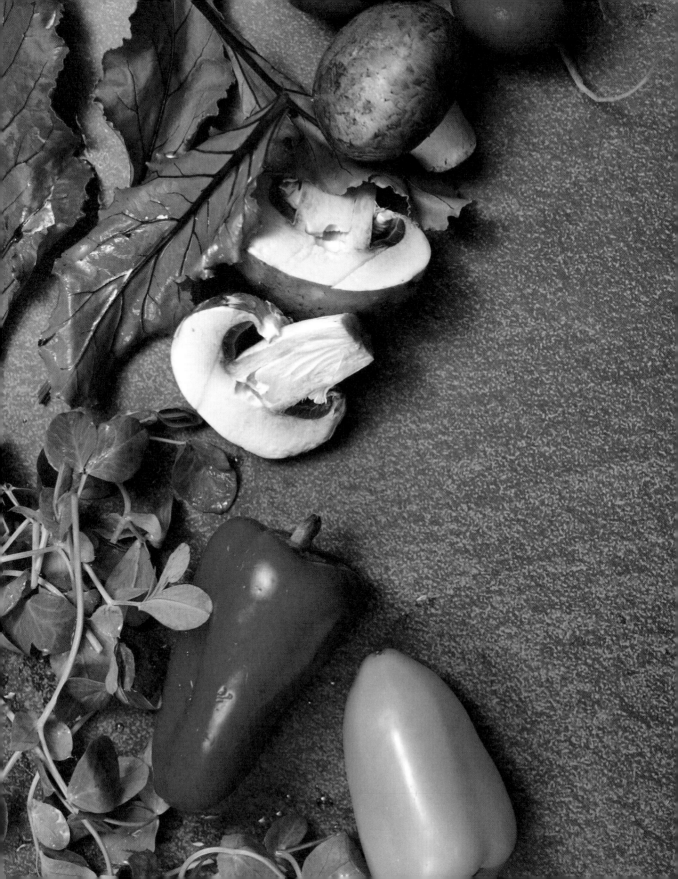

CHAPTER 10

SECRET SAUCES

Spicy Green Goddess Dressing

Prep Time: 5 minutes
Cook Time: None
Yield: 1½ cups

This blend of fresh herbs, hot jalapeño, and creamy tahini is a twist on the traditional green goddess dressing. Serve as a dip with Crispy Smashed Fingerling Potatoes (page 115) or crudité, or drizzle over your favorite salad.

1 cup roughly chopped fresh chives
1 cup roughly chopped fresh cilantro
1 jalapeño, deseeded and roughly chopped
2 garlic cloves
4 tbsp tahini
4 tbsp nutritional yeast
2 tbsp miso paste
4 tbsp freshly squeezed lime juice
⅔ cup water
1 tbsp chia seeds

1. In a blender, purée the chives, cilantro, jalapeño, and garlic cloves for 30 to 60 seconds. Add the tahini, nutritional yeast, miso paste, lime juice, water, and chia seeds. Blend until smooth.

2. Serve immediately, or store in an airtight container in the refrigerator for up to 4 or 5 days.

Balsamic-Tahini Dressing

Prep Time: 5 minutes
Cook Time: None
Yield: ½ cup

An amazing health-forward version of a vinaigrette, this recipe uses tahini to enhance sweet-and-tangy balsamic vinegar, making a creamy, decadent dressing.

4 tbsp balsamic glaze
2 tbsp tahini
1 tsp minced fresh ginger
1 tsp minced garlic
3–4 tbsp water to thin, as desired

1. In a medium bowl, whisk together all dressing ingredients until well combined.

2. Serve immediately, or store in an airtight container in the refrigerator for up to 6 days.

Russian Dressing

Prep Time: 5 minutes
Cook Time: None
Yield: ¾ cup

Seven simple staples are combined for a nutritious take on Russian dressing. Perfect for the Tempeh Reuben Salad (page 136) or any other salad you prefer. Double or triple the recipe to have it on hand during the week.

¼ cup raw cashews
2 tbsp ketchup
2 tbsp apple cider
   vinegar
1 tbsp dill relish
1 tsp onion powder
1 tsp freshly ground
   black pepper
¼ cup plant milk

1. To a high-speed blender, add all dressing ingredients, and blend until smooth.

2. Serve immediately, or store in an airtight container in the refrigerator for up to 5 days.

Cilantro-Lime Dressing

Instead of nuts or seeds as a base, this enlightened dressing uses creamy, fiber-rich cannellini beans. The classic combo of cilantro and lime is perfect in this balanced blend to use as a companion over any recipe that can welcome some additional fresh fabulousness.

1 (15oz; 425g) can low-sodium cannellini beans, drained and rinsed

½ cup chopped fresh cilantro

¼ cup nutritional yeast

2 tbsp tahini

2 tbsp reduced-sodium tamari

2 tbsp freshly squeezed lime juice

1 tbsp maple syrup

⅛ tsp red pepper flakes

½ cup plant milk

1. To a high-speed blender, add all dressing ingredients, and blend until smooth.

2. Serve immediately, or store in an airtight container in the refrigerator for up to 5 days.

Hemp Seed Ranch Dressing

Prep Time: 5 minutes
Cook Time: None
Yield: 1 cup

This fresh version of ranch dressing features plenty of herbs and exquisite nutrition, with omega-3s in the hemp seeds, phytonutrients in the greens, and a hint of acid to help your body absorb the minerals from the dressing itself and any greens you serve with it.

½ cup hemp seeds
2 tbsp nutritional yeast
2 tbsp chopped
   fresh dill
2 tbsp chopped
   fresh chives
1 tbsp chopped fresh
   flat-leaf parsley
2½ tsp apple cider
   vinegar
1½ tsp freshly squeezed
   lemon juice
1 tsp anchovy-free
   Worcestershire sauce
1 tsp onion powder
1 tsp garlic powder
¼ tsp freshly ground
   black pepper
½ cup plant milk

1. To a high-speed blender, add all dressing ingredients, and blend until smooth.

2. Serve immediately, or store in an airtight container in the refrigerator for up to 5 days.

Prep Time: 15 minutes

Cook Time: 1 minute

Yield: 1½ cups

Almond Tzatziki Whip

Almonds offer a unique, grainy texture when blanched and puréed. Together with fresh cucumber and dill, and a splash of vibrant acid, this is a balanced topper that can be used as a dressing or dip.

½ cup raw almonds

½ English cucumber, peeled and shredded (about 1 cup), divided

3 cloves garlic, sliced

2 tbsp chopped fresh dill

1 tbsp freshly squeezed lemon juice

1 tbsp apple cider vinegar

1 tbsp reduced-sodium tamari

¼ tsp freshly ground black pepper

1. In a small saucepan, bring 2 cups water to a boil. Add the almonds, and boil for 1 minute. Drain and shock with cold water. Using your fingers, gently squeeze to remove the skins. Discard skins.

2. To a high-powered blender, add the blanched almonds, ½ cup cucumber, garlic, dill, lemon juice, apple cider vinegar, tamari, and pepper. Blend until smooth. Add the remaining ½ cup cucumber, and pulse once or twice. Serve immediately, or store in an airtight container in the refrigerator for up 5 days.

Carrot-Ginger Dressing

Prep Time: 10 minutes
Cook Time: None
Yield: 3½ cups

Transform any plain salad into a vibrant, bright, zesty delight with this delicious dressing. Inspired by Japanese restaurant-style green salad, you can be certain to pile up the veggies when this is the topper.

2 cups sliced carrot
1 celery stalk, chopped
¼ cup chopped apple
¼ cup peeled and chopped orange
1 small shallot, chopped
1 tbsp tahini
1 tbsp minced fresh ginger
1 tbsp reduced-sodium tamari
½ tbsp miso paste
¼ cup rice wine vinegar
¼ cup plant milk
½ tsp freshly ground black pepper, or more to taste

1. To a blender, add all ingredients, and blend until smooth.

2. Serve immediately, or store in an airtight container in the refrigerator for up to 5 days.

Prep Time: 10 minutes
Cook Time: None
Yield: 2 cups

Cilantro-Mint Sauce

A unique play on chutney, this sauce combines fresh herbs and a bit of heat from jalapeño. White beans give it a hearty texture that is super satisfying. Enjoy with **Potato-Pea Samosa Patties (page 108)** or crudité.

1 (15oz; 425g) can Great Northern beans (or cannellini or other white beans), drained and rinsed

1 cup chopped fresh cilantro

¼ cup chopped fresh mint

2 scallions, chopped

2 tbsp freshly squeezed lemon juice

1 tbsp chopped jalapeño

1 tsp miso paste

½ tsp garlic powder

½ tsp ground cumin

½ cup water

1. To a blender, add all ingredients, and blend until smooth.

2. Serve immediately, or store in an airtight container in the refrigerator for up to 5 days.

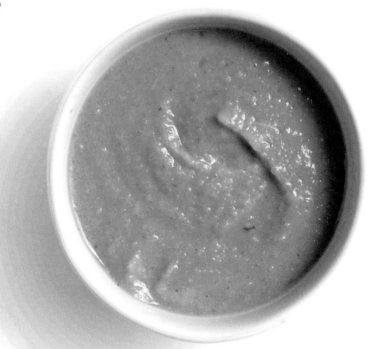

Spicy Peanut Dipping Sauce

Prep Time: 5 minutes
Cook Time: None
Yield: ¾ cup

This is my go-to template for spicy peanut sauce. You can modify according to your preferences—use less hot sauce if you prefer mild heat, add more vinegar or lime if you like a bit more acid, or toss in freshly roasted peanuts hot out of the oven. Experiment until you find your perfect version!

¼ cup natural peanut butter (no added salt, sugar, or stabilizers)

2 tbsp rice wine vinegar

2 tbsp freshly squeezed lime or lemon juice

2 tsp minced fresh ginger

1–2 tbsp sriracha or other hot sauce

1 tsp reduced-sodium tamari

1 tsp maple syrup

1–2 tbsp water, to desired consistency

1. To a blender, add all ingredients, and blend until smooth.

2. Serve immediately with Korean Summer Rolls (page 118) or raw veggies, or store in an airtight container in the refrigerator for up to 4 days.

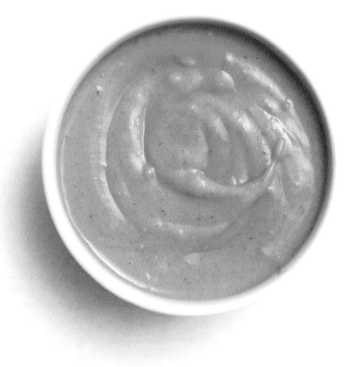

Prep Time: 10 minutes +
roasting garlic

Cook Time: None

Yield: 3½ cups

Spinach Artichoke Hummus

Hummus should be a food group, as I always say! This briny, green, flavorful variety validates this claim and adds to a simple, savvy repertoire of bean-based dips to enjoy with crudité, over salad, with a spoon, or however you love to hummus.

2 (15oz; 425g) cans chickpeas

1 cup artichoke hearts in brine, drained

3 tbsp nutritional yeast

3 tbsp freshly squeezed lemon juice

2 tbsp tahini

2 tbsp reduced-sodium tamari

6 or more roasted garlic cloves (see note)

1 tsp dry mustard powder (ground mustard)

1 tsp freshly ground black pepper

6oz (170g) baby spinach

1 tsp red pepper flakes (optional; or use lemon pepper or paprika), to garnish

1. Drain the chickpeas, reserving ½ cup aquafaba (liquid from chickpea can).

2. To a food processor, add the chickpeas, ½ cup aquafaba, artichoke hearts, nutritional yeast, lemon juice, tahini, tamari, garlic, mustard powder, and pepper. Blend until well combined. Stop and scrape the walls, and blend again for 15 to 20 seconds. Add the spinach, and pulse until spinach is incorporated but not fully broken down.

3. Sprinkle with red pepper flakes, if using. Serve immediately with crudité, with a salad, or over a baked potato.

NOTE Raw garlic can be used, but roasting brings out sweetness and flavor. To make roasted garlic, wrap 1 whole garlic bulb in foil and roast in a 375°F (190°C) oven for 30 minutes or until soft.

Harissa Butternut Squash Hummus

Prep Time: 10 minutes
Cook Time: None
Yield: 3½ cups

With only seven staple ingredients, you can whip up a batch of hummus anytime for friends or family—or keep it all to yourself if you are a hummus lover like me. Butternut squash adds a bright, carotenoid complexion (pun intended, as carotenoids are excellent for the skin), and the harissa and chipotle combo is wonderfully warm.

2 (15oz; 425g) cans chickpeas

1 cup baked butternut squash, flesh only (or use canned purée)

2 tbsp freshly squeezed lemon juice

2 tbsp tahini

1 tbsp reduced-sodium tamari

2 tbsp ground harissa seasoning

1 tsp chipotle powder

1. Drain the chickpeas, reserving ¾ cup aquafaba (liquid from 1 can of chickpeas). To a food processor, add the chickpeas, reserved aquafaba, butternut squash, lemon juice, tahini, tamari, harissa, and chipotle powder. Purée until smooth.

2. Serve with crudité or whole-grain crackers, and store in the refrigerator in an airtight container to up to 5 days.

Prep Time: 10 minutes
Cook Time: 45–60 minutes
Yield: 8 cups

Simple Marinara Sauce

There are many commercially available marinara sauces, but they almost always have excessive sugars, oils, salts, and preservatives. Fortunately, marinara sauce is surprisingly simple to DIY at home, and it need not be complicated. Here is a super-simple template to try. Cook this up, adding or removing seasonings, as desired. Store it in Mason jars, and use with vegetables, noodles, or Spaghetti (Squash) Lasagna (page 94).

2 cups diced yellow onion
4–6 cloves garlic, minced
2 (28oz; 794g) cans low-sodium crushed tomatoes
1 (6oz; 170g) can tomato paste
1 tsp dried basil
1 tsp dried oregano
1 bay leaf
1 tbsp maple syrup
¼–½ tsp red pepper flakes, to taste
Freshly ground black pepper (optional), to taste

1. Heat a large saucepan or Dutch oven over medium-high heat. When hot, sauté the onion with as little water as possible, just enough to avoid burning, for 4 to 6 minutes until beginning to brown. Add the garlic, and cook for 1 minute more.

2. Add the tomatoes, tomato paste, basil, oregano, bay leaf, maple syrup, and red pepper flakes. Stir to combine, and bring to a boil. Reduce the heat, cover, and simmer for 45 to 60 minutes, stirring occasionally. (It will thicken with time.)

3. Remove from the heat, and remove the bay leaf. Season with pepper, if desired. Serve immediately, or allow to cool and refrigerate in an airtight container for up to 5 days.

Sweet Potato Cheesy Sauce

Prep Time: 10 minutes
Cook Time: 40–60 minutes
Yield: 5 cups

Yet another tasty treat you can make with the super-versatile potato. Add some reliable nooch, and this sweet potato becomes a queso that is creamy, flavorful, and filling. Use it for a healthy mac 'n' cheese (page 80), as a topping for veggies, or any way you enjoy a creamy, cheesy queso.

2 sweet potatoes
½ cup raw cashews
4 tbsp nutritional yeast
1 tsp dry mustard powder
½ tsp garlic powder
½ tsp onion powder
½ tsp chipotle powder
½ tsp smoked paprika
2 tbsp freshly squeezed lemon juice
1 tbsp reduced-sodium tamari
2 cups plant milk

1. Preheat the oven to 400°F (200°C). Line a baking sheet with a silicone baking mat or parchment paper. Scrub the potatoes well and poke holes in the flesh a few times with a fork. Place on the prepared baking sheet, and bake for 40 to 60 minutes or until juices begin to seep out and the potatoes are easily pierced with a toothpick or knife.

2. When cool, scoop the potato flesh from the skin and place in a high-speed blender. Add the cashews, nutritional yeast, mustard powder, garlic powder, onion powder, chipotle powder, smoked paprika, lemon juice, tamari, and plant milk. Blend until smooth.

3. Serve immediately, or store in an airtight container in the refrigerator for up to 5 days.

Spicy Cashew Cheesy Sauce

Prep Time: 5 minutes
Cook Time: None
Yield: 1½ cups

A simple, balanced, and picante queso sauce made with pantry staples that can spice up a salad, a baked potato, or veggies. Bright and creamy, this is a go-to option you can quickly whip up anytime.

½ cup raw cashews
½ cup roasted red pepper (jarred in water)
4–5 tbsp nutritional yeast flakes
2 tbsp freshly squeezed lemon juice
1 tbsp reduced-sodium tamari
1 tsp maple syrup
¼–½ tsp cayenne
¼ cup plant milk

1. To a high-speed blender, add all ingredients, and blend on high until smooth.

2. Serve immediately as a dip or sauce, or store in an airtight container in the refrigerator for up to 5 days.

Nacho Squash Sauce

Prep Time: 10 minutes
Cook Time: 40 minutes
Yield: 4 cups

A play on cashew queso with some extra-spicy pizazz! The starch from the potato adds ooey-gooey texture, and the squash provides a vibrant color. Enjoy over steamed veggies or a baked potato.

1 small butternut squash
1 Yukon Gold potato
1 (4oz; 113g) can green chiles
½ cup raw cashews
½ cup nutritional yeast
2 tbsp freshly squeezed lemon juice
1 tbsp reduced-sodium tamari
1 tbsp chili powder
1 tsp chipotle powder
½ tsp cayenne
1½ cups plant milk

1. Preheat the oven to 375°F (190°C). Line a baking sheet with parchment paper or a silicone baking mat. Place the whole butternut squash and potato on the prepared baking sheet, and roast for 40 minutes or until the skin of the squash is brown and bubbling.

2. When cool enough to handle, cut the squash in half lengthwise, remove the seeds, and scoop out the flesh. Measure out 2 cups cooked squash, and place in a high-speed blender. (Reserve any additional squash for another use.)

3. To the blender, add the cooked potato, green chiles, cashews, nutritional yeast, lemon juice, tamari, chili powder, chipotle powder, cayenne, and plant milk. Blend on high until smooth.

4. Serve immediately as a dip or sauce, or store in an airtight container in the refrigerator for up to 5 days.

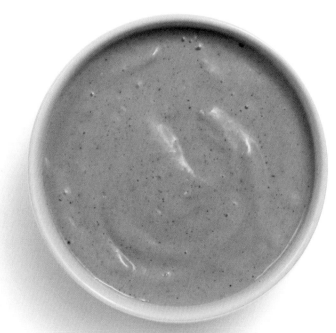

Endnotes

Introduction

1 "Adult Obesity Facts." Centers for Disease Control and Prevention. Centers for Disease Control and Prevention, February 11, 2021. https://www.cdc.gov/obesity/data/adult.html.

2 "Obesity and Overweight." World Health Organization. World Health Organization. Accessed April 22, 2021. https://www.who.int/news-room/fact-sheets/detail/obesity-and-overweight.

Chapter 1

1 Hamwi, George J. "Therapy: changing dietary concepts." Diabetes mellitus: diagnosis and treatment 1 (1964): 73-78.

Chapter 2

1 Turner-McGrievy, Gabrielle, Trisha Mandes, and Anthony Crimarco. "A plant-based diet for overweight and obesity prevention and treatment." Journal of geriatric cardiology: JGC 14, no. 5 (2017): 369.

2 Turner-McGrievy, Gabrielle M., Charis R. Davidson, Ellen E. Wingard, Sara Wilcox, and Edward A. Frongillo. "Comparative effectiveness of plant-based diets for weight loss: a randomized controlled trial of five different diets." Nutrition 31, no. 2 (2015): 350-358.

3 Brownlee, Iain A., Peter I. Chater, Jeff P. Pearson, and Matt D. Wilcox. "Dietary fibre and weight loss: Where are we now?." Food Hydrocolloids 68 (2017): 186-191.

4 Afshin, Ashkan, Patrick John Sur, Kairsten A. Fay, Leslie Cornaby, Giannina Ferrara, Joseph S. Salama, Erin C. Mullany et al. "Health effects of dietary risks in 195 countries, 1990–2017: a systematic analysis for the Global Burden of Disease Study 2017." The Lancet 393, no. 10184 (2019): 1958-1972.

5 Ornish, Dean, Larry W. Scherwitz, James H. Billings, K. Lance Gould, Terri A. Merritt, Stephen Sparler, William T. Armstrong et al. "Intensive lifestyle changes for reversal of coronary heart disease." Jama 280, no. 23 (1998): 2001-2007.

6 Esselstyn Jr, Caldwell B., Gina Gendy, Jonathan Doyle, Mladen Golubic, and Michael F. Roizen. "A way to reverse CAD?." Journal of Family Practice 63, no. 7 (2014): 356-364.

7 Barnard, Neal D., Joshua Cohen, David JA Jenkins, Gabrielle Turner-McGrievy, Lise Gloede, Amber Green, and Hope Ferdowsian. "A low-fat vegan diet and a conventional diabetes diet in the treatment of type 2 diabetes: a randomized, controlled, 74-wk clinical trial." The American journal of clinical nutrition 89, no. 5 (2009): 1588S-1596S.

8 Yokoyama, Yoko, Neal D. Barnard, Susan M. Levin, and Mitsuhiro Watanabe. "Vegetarian diets and glycemic control in diabetes: a systematic review and meta-analysis." Cardiovascular diagnosis and therapy 4, no. 5 (2014): 373.

9 Kim, Hyunju, Laura E. Caulfield, Vanessa Garcia☐Larsen, Lyn M. Steffen, Josef Coresh, and Casey M. Rebholz. "Plant☐Based diets are associated with a lower risk of incident cardiovascular disease, cardiovascular disease mortality, and All☐Cause mortality in a general population of Middle☐Aged adults." Journal of the American Heart Association 8, no. 16 (2019): e012865.

10 Orlich, Michael J., Pramil N. Singh, Joan Sabaté, Karen Jaceldo-Siegl, Jing Fan, Synnove Knutsen, W. Lawrence Beeson, and Gary E. Fraser. "Vegetarian dietary patterns and mortality in Adventist Health Study 2." JAMA internal medicine 173, no. 13 (2013): 1230-1238.

11 Wang, Dong, Yanping Li, Yuk-Lam Ho, Xuan-Mai Nguyen, Rebecca J. Song, Frank B. Hu, Walter Willett et al. "Plant-Based Diet and the Risk of Cardiovascular Disease and Mortality: The Million Veteran Program." Current Developments in Nutrition 4, no. Supplement_2 (2020): 1502-1502.

12 Pettersen, Betty J., Ramtin Anousheh, Jing Fan, Karen Jaceldo-Siegl, and Gary E. Fraser. "Vegetarian diets and blood pressure among white subjects: results from the Adventist Health Study-2 (AHS-2)." Public health nutrition 15, no. 10 (2012): 1909-1916.

13 Jenkins, David JA, Cyril WC Kendall, Augustine Marchie, Dorothea A. Faulkner, Julia MW Wong, Russell de Souza, Azadeh Emam et al. "Direct comparison of a dietary portfolio of cholesterol-lowering foods with a statin in hypercholesterolemic participants." The American journal of clinical nutrition 81, no. 2 (2005): 380-387.

14 Rosell, M., P. Appleby, E. Spencer, and T. Key. "Weight gain over 5 years in 21 966 meat-eating, fish-eating, vegetarian, and vegan men and women in EPIC-Oxford." International journal of obesity 30, no. 9 (2006): 1389-1396.

15 Wang, Youfa, and May A. Beydoun. "Meat consumption is associated with obesity and central obesity among US adults." International journal of obesity 33, no. 6 (2009): 621-628.

16 Tonstad, Serena, Terry Butler, Ru Yan, and Gary E. Fraser. "Type of vegetarian diet, body weight, and prevalence of type 2 diabetes." Diabetes care 32, no. 5 (2009): 791-796.

17 Hever, Julieanna. "Plant-based diets: A physician's guide." The permanente journal 20, no. 3 (2016).

18 Hever, Julieanna, and Raymond J. Cronise. "Plant-based nutrition for healthcare professionals: implementing diet as a primary modality in the prevention and treatment of chronic disease." Journal of geriatric cardiology: JGC 14, no. 5 (2017): 355.

19 Eyres, Laurence, Michael F. Eyres, Alexandra Chisholm, and Rachel C. Brown. "Coconut oil consumption and cardiovascular risk factors in humans." Nutrition reviews 74, no. 4 (2016): 267-280.

20 American Heart Association. "Shaking the salt habit to lower high blood pressure." (2017).

21 Davis, Caroline, and Jacqueline C. Carter. "If certain foods are addictive, how might this change the treatment of compulsive overeating and obesity?." Current addiction reports 1, no. 2 (2014): 89-95.

22 Miura, Hirohito, and Linda A. Barlow. "Taste bud regeneration and the search for taste progenitor cells." Archives italiennes de biologie 148, no. 2 (2010): 107.

23 Beidler, Lloyd M., and Ronald L. Smallman. "Renewal of cells within taste buds." Journal of Cell Biology 27, no. 2 (1965): 263-272.

24 Willett, Walter C. "The Mediterranean diet: science and practice." Public health nutrition 9, no. 1a (2006): 105-110.

25 Davis, Courtney, Janet Bryan, Jonathan Hodgson, and Karen Murphy. "Definition of the Mediterranean diet; a literature review." Nutrients 7, no. 11 (2015): 9139-9153.

26 Willcox, Donald Craig, Giovanni Scapagnini, and Bradley J. Willcox. "Healthy aging diets other than the Mediterranean: a focus on the Okinawan diet." Mechanisms of ageing and development 136 (2014): 148-162.

27 Willcox, D. Craig, Bradley J. Willcox, Hidemi Todoriki, and Makoto Suzuki. "The Okinawan diet: health implications of a low-calorie, nutrient-dense, antioxidant-rich dietary pattern low in glycemic load." Journal of the American College of Nutrition 28, no. sup4 (2009): 500S-516S.

28 Barnard, Neal D., Jihad Alwarith, Emilie Rembert, Liz Brandon, Minh Nguyen, Andrea Goergen, Taylor Horne et al. "A Mediterranean diet and low-fat vegan diet to improve body weight and cardiometabolic risk factors: A randomized, cross-over trial." Journal of the American College of Nutrition (2020): 1-13.

29 Jenkins, David JA, Julia MW Wong, Cyril WC Kendall, Amin Esfahani, Vivian WY Ng, Tracy CK Leong, Dorothea A. Faulkner et al. "Effect of a 6-month vegan low-carbohydrate ('Eco-Atkins') diet on cardiovascular risk factors and body weight in hyperlipidaemic adults: a randomised controlled trial." BMJ open 4, no. 2 (2014).

30 Seidelmann, Sara B., Brian Claggett, Susan Cheng, Mir Henglin, Amil Shah, Lyn M. Steffen, Aaron R. Folsom, Eric B. Rimm, Walter C. Willett, and Scott D. Solomon. "Dietary carbohydrate intake and mortality: a prospective cohort study and meta-analysis." The Lancet Public Health 3, no. 9 (2018): e419-e428.

31 Festi, D., A. Colecchia, M. Orsini, A. Sangermano, S. Sottili, P. Simoni, G. Mazzella et al. "Gallbladder motility and gallstone formation in obese patients following very low calorie diets. Use it (fat) to lose it (well)." International journal of obesity 22, no. 6 (1998): 592-600.

32 Del Gobbo, Liana C., Michael C. Falk, Robin Feldman, Kara Lewis, and Dariush Mozaffarian. "Effects of tree nuts on blood lipids, apolipoproteins, and blood pressure: systematic review, meta-analysis, and dose-response of 61 controlled intervention trials." The American journal of clinical nutrition 102, no. 6 (2015): 1347-1356.

33 Ros, Emilio. "Nuts and novel biomarkers of cardiovascular disease." The American journal of clinical nutrition 89, no. 5 (2009): 1649S-1656S.

34 Natoli, Sharon, and Penelope McCoy. "A review of the evidence: nuts and body weight." Asia Pacific journal of clinical nutrition 16, no. 4 (2007).

35 Tan, Sze Yen, Jaapna Dhillon, and Richard D. Mattes. "A review of the effects of nuts on appetite, food intake, metabolism, and body weight." The American journal of clinical nutrition 100, no. suppl_1 (2014):412S-422S.

36 Rajaram, Sujatha, and Joan Sabaté. "Nuts, body weight and insulin resistance." British Journal of Nutrition 96, no. S2 (2006): S79-S86.

37 Mattes, Richard D., Penny M. Kris-Etherton, and Gary D. Foster. "Impact of peanuts and tree nuts on body weight and healthy weight loss in adults." The Journal of nutrition 138, no. 9 (2008): 1741S-1745S.

38 Mattes, Richard D., and Mark L. Dreher. "Nuts and healthy body weight maintenance mechanisms." Asia Pacific journal of clinical nutrition 19, no. 1 (2010): 137.

39 Tindall, Alyssa M., Emily A. Johnston, Penny M. Kris-Etherton, and Kristina S. Petersen. "The effect of nuts on markers of glycemic control: a systematic review and meta-analysis of randomized controlled trials." The American journal of clinical nutrition 109, no. 2 (2019): 297-314.

40 Guarneiri, Liana L., and Jamie A. Cooper. "Intake of nuts or nut products does not lead to weight gain, independent of dietary substitution instructions: A systematic review and meta-analysis of randomized trials." Advances in Nutrition 12, no. 2 (2021): 384-401.

41 Duarte, Patrícia Fonseca, Marcia Alves Chaves, Caroline Dellinghausen Borges, and Carla Rosane Barboza Mendonça. "Avocado: characteristics, health benefits and uses." Ciência Rural 46, no. 4 (2016): 747-754.

42 Peou, Sokunthea, Brittany Milliard-Hasting, and Sachin A. Shah. "Impact of avocado-enriched diets on plasma lipoproteins: a meta-analysis." Journal of clinical lipidology 10, no. 1 (2016): 161-171.

43 Fulgoni, Victor L., Mark Dreher, and Adrienne J. Davenport. "Avocado consumption is associated with better diet quality and nutrient intake, and lower metabolic syndrome risk in US adults: results from the National Health and Nutrition Examination Survey (NHANES) 2001–2008." Nutrition journal 12, no. 1 (2013): 1-6.

44 Messina, Mark. "Soy and health update: evaluation of the clinical and epidemiologic literature." Nutrients 8, no. 12 (2016): 754.

45 Blanco Mejia, Sonia, Mark Messina, Siying S. Li, Effie Viguiliouk, Laura Chiavaroli, Tauseef A. Khan, Korbua Srichaikul et al. "A meta-analysis of 46 studies identified by the FDA demonstrates that soy protein decreases circulating LDL and total cholesterol concentrations in adults." The Journal of nutrition 149, no. 6 (2019): 968-981.

46 Jenkins, David JA, Sonia Blanco Mejia, Laura Chiavaroli, Effie Viguiliouk, Siying S. Li, Cyril WC Kendall, Vladmir Vuksan, and John L. Sievenpiper. "Cumulative meta☐analysis of the soy effect over time." Journal of the American Heart Association 8, no. 13 (2019): e012458.

47 Blanco Mejia, Sonia, Mark Messina, Siying S. Li, Effie Viguiliouk, Laura Chiavaroli, Tauseef A. Khan, Korbua Srichaikul et al. "A meta-analysis of 46 studies identified by the FDA demonstrates that soy protein decreases circulating LDL and total cholesterol concentrations in adults." The Journal of nutrition 149, no. 6 (2019): 968-981.

48 Wilde, Peter J. "Eating for life: designing foods for appetite control." Journal of diabetes science and technology 3, no. 2 (2009): 366-370.

49 Hargrave, Sara L., and Kimberly P. Kinzig. "Repeated gastric distension alters food intake and neuroendocrine profiles in rats." Physiology & behavior 105, no. 4 (2012): 975-981.

50 Regmi, Prashant, and Leonie K. Heilbronn. "Time Restricted eating: Benefits, Mechanisms, and Challenges in Translation." Iscience (2020): 101161.

51 Wilkinson, Michael J., Emily NC Manoogian, Adena Zadourian, Hannah Lo, Savannah Fakhouri, Azarin Shoghi, Xinran Wang et al. "Ten-hour time-restricted eating reduces weight, blood pressure, and atherogenic lipids in patients with metabolic syndrome." Cell metabolism 31, no. 1 (2020): 92-104.

52 Moon, Shinje, Jiseung Kang, Sang Hyun Kim, Hye Soo Chung, Yoon Jung Kim, Jae Myung Yu, Sung Tae Cho, Chang-Myung Oh, and Tae Kim. "Beneficial effects of time-restricted eating on metabolic diseases: a systemic review and meta-analysis." Nutrients 12, no. 5 (2020): 1267.

53 Longo, Valter D., and Satchidananda Panda. "Fasting, circadian rhythms, and time-restricted feeding in healthy lifespan." Cell metabolism 23, no. 6 (2016): 1048-1059.

54 Kvietys, P. R. "Postprandial hyperemia." The Gastrointestinal Circulation. San Rafael, CA: Morgan & Claypool Life Sciences (2010).

55 Jia, Guanghong, and James R. Sowers. "Autophagy: a housekeeper in cardiorenal metabolic health and disease." Biochimica et Biophysica Acta (BBA)-Molecular Basis of Disease 1852, no. 2 (2015): 219-224.

56 Raynor, Hollie A. "Can limiting dietary variety assist with reducing energy intake and weight loss?." Physiology & behavior 106, no. 3 (2012): 356-361.

57 Raynor, Hollie A., Robert W. Jeffery, Suzanne Phelan, James O. Hill, and Rena R. Wing. "Amount of food group variety consumed in the diet and long☐term weight loss maintenance." Obesity research 13, no. 5 (2005): 883-890.

Chapter 5

1   Martin, Crescent B., Kirsten A. Herrick, Neda Sarafrazi, and Cynthia L. Ogden. Attempts to lose weight among adults in the United States, 2013-2016. US Department of Health and Human Services, Centers for Disease Control and Prevention, National Center for Health Statistics, 2018.

2   Hall, Kevin D., and Scott Kahan. "Maintenance of lost weight and long-term management of obesity." Medical Clinics 102, no. 1 (2018): 183-197.

3   Varkevisser, R. D. M., M. M. van Stralen, W. Kroeze, J. C. F. Ket, and I. H. M. Steenhuis. "Determinants of weight loss maintenance: a systematic review." Obesity reviews 20, no. 2 (2019): 171-211.

4   Neumann, Maria, Christina Holzapfel, Astrid Müller, Anja Hilbert, Ross D. Crosby, and Martina de Zwaan. "Features and trajectories of eating behavior in weight☐loss maintenance: results from the German Weight Control Registry." Obesity 26, no. 9 (2018): 1501-1508.

5   Butryn, Meghan L., Suzanne Phelan, James O. Hill, and Rena R. Wing. "Consistent self☐monitoring of weight: a key component of successful weight loss maintenance." Obesity 15, no. 12 (2007): 3091-3096.

6   Kruger, Judy, Heidi Michels Blanck, and Cathleen Gillespie. "Dietary and physical activity behaviors among adults successful at weight loss maintenance." International Journal of Behavioral Nutrition and Physical Activity 3, no. 1 (2006): 1-10.

7   Paixão, Catarina, Carlos M. Dias, Rui Jorge, Eliana V. Carraça, Mary Yannakoulia, Martina de Zwaan, Sirpa Soini, James O. Hill, Pedro J. Teixeira, and Inês Santos. "Successful weight loss maintenance: a systematic review of weight control registries." Obesity Reviews 21, no. 5 (2020): e13003.

8   Manchali, Shivapriya, Kotamballi N. Chidambara Murthy, and Bhimanagouda S. Patil. "Crucial facts about health benefits of popular cruciferous vegetables." Journal of functional foods 4, no. 1 (2012): 94-106.

9   Abdull Razis, Ahmad Faizal, and Noramaliza Mohd Noor. "Cruciferous vegetables: dietary phytochemicals for cancer prevention." Asian Pacific Journal of cancer prevention 14, no. 3 (2013): 1565-1570.

10 Santín-Márquez, Roberto, Adriana Alarcón-Aguilar, Norma Edith López-Diazguerrero, Niki Chondrogianni, and Mina Königsberg. "Sulforaphane-role in aging and neurodegeneration." GeroScience 41, no. 5 (2019): 655-670.

11 Bsc, Sc Noonan, and Gp Savage Bsc. "Oxalate content of foods and its effect on humans." Asia Pacific journal of clinical nutrition 8, no. 1 (1999): 64-74.

12 Natesh, H. N., L. Abbey, and S. K. Asiedu. "An overview of nutritional and antinutritional factors in green leafy vegetables." Horticult Int J 1, no. 2 (2017): 00011.

13 Imodaifer, Shuruq, Noura Alsibaie, G. Alhoumendan, Ghadeer Alammari, and M. S. Kavita. "Role of phytochemicals in health and nutrition." BAO J Nutr 3 (2017): 28-34.

14 Milani, Alireza, Marzieh Basirnejad, Sepideh Shahbazi, and Azam Bolhassani. "Carotenoids: biochemistry, pharmacology and treatment." British journal of pharmacology 174, no. 11 (2017): 1290-1324.

15 Wan, Qianyi, Ni Li, Liang Du, Rui Zhao, Mengshi Yi, Qiushi Xu, and Yong Zhou. "Allium vegetable consumption and health: An umbrella review of meta☐analyses of multiple health outcomes." Food science & nutrition 7, no. 8 (2019): 2451-2470.

16 Kothari, Damini, Woo-Do Lee, and Soo-Ki Kim. "Allium Flavonols: Health Benefits, Molecular Targets, and Bioavailability." Antioxidants 9, no. 9 (2020): 888.

17 Torres-Palazzolo, Carolina, Daniela Ramirez, Daniela Locatelli, Walter Manucha, Claudia Castro, and Alejandra Camargo. "Bioaccessibility and permeability of bioactive compounds in raw and cooked garlic." Journal of Food Composition and Analysis 70 (2018): 49-53.

18 Frankel, Farrell, Matthew Priven, Elizabeth Richard, Chloe Schweinshault, Oni Tongo, Abrielle Webster, Elizabeth Barth, Kristen Slejzer, and Sari Edelstein. "Health functionality of organosulfides: a review." International Journal of Food Properties 19, no. 3 (2016): 537-548.

19 Lee, Yoon-Mi, Young Yoon, Haelim Yoon, Hyun-Min Park, Sooji Song, and Kyung-Jin Yeum. "Dietary anthocyanins against obesity and inflammation." Nutrients 9, no. 10 (2017): 1089.

20 Tian, Lingmin, Yisha Tan, Guowei Chen, Gang Wang, Jianxia Sun, Shiyi Ou, Wei Chen, and Weibin Bai. "Metabolism of anthocyanins and consequent effects on the gut microbiota." Critical reviews in food science and nutrition 59, no. 6 (2019): 982-991.

21 Sharif, Niloufar, Sara Khoshnoudi-Nia, and Seid Mahdi Jafari. "Nano/microencapsulation of anthocyanins; a systematic review and meta-analysis." Food Research International 132 (2020): 109077.

22 Khoo, Hock Eng, Azrina Azlan, Sou Teng Tang, and See Meng Lim. "Anthocyanidins and anthocyanins: colored pigments as food, pharmaceutical ingredients, and the potential health benefits." Food & nutrition research 61, no. 1 (2017): 1361779.

23 World Health Organization. "Increasing fruit and vegetable consumption to reduce the risk of noncommunicable diseases." WHO: Geneva, Switzerland (2014).

24 Natoli, Sharon, and Penelope McCoy. "A review of the evidence: nuts and body weight." Asia Pacific journal of clinical nutrition 16, no. 4 (2007).

25 Soeliman, Fatemeh Azizi, and Leila Azadbakht. "Weight loss maintenance: A review on dietary related strategies." Journal of research in medical sciences: the official journal of Isfahan University of Medical Sciences 19, no. 3 (2014): 268.

26 St-Onge, Marie-Pierre. "Dietary fats, teas, dairy, and nuts: potential functional foods for weight control?." The American journal of clinical nutrition 81, no. 1 (2005): 7-15.

27 Karfopoulou, Eleni, Dora Brikou, Eirini Mamalaki, Fragiskos Bersimis, Costas A. Anastasiou, James O. Hill, and Mary Yannakoulia. "Dietary patterns in weight loss maintenance: results from the MedWeight study." European journal of nutrition 56, no. 3 (2017): 991-1002.

28 Li, Zhaoping, Rubens Song, Christine Nguyen, Alona Zerlin, Hannah Karp, Kris Naowamondhol, Gail Thames et al. "Pistachio nuts reduce triglycerides and body weight by comparison to refined carbohydrate snack in obese subjects on a 12-week weight loss program." Journal of the American College of Nutrition 29, no. 3 (2010): 198-203.

29 Tan, Sze Yen, Jaapna Dhillon, and Richard D. Mattes. "A review of the effects of nuts on appetite, food intake, metabolism, and body weight." The American journal of clinical nutrition 100, no. suppl_1 (2014): 412S-422S.

30 Freitas, Jullyana Borges, and Maria Margareth Veloso Naves. "Chemical composition of nuts and edible seeds and their relation to nutrition and health." Revista de Nutrição 23, no. 2 (2010): 269-279.

31 Tindall, Alyssa M., Emily A. Johnston, Penny M. Kris-Etherton, and Kristina S. Petersen. "The effect of nuts on markers of glycemic control: a systematic review and meta-analysis of randomized controlled trials." The American journal of clinical nutrition 109, no. 2 (2019): 297-314.

32 Aune, Dagfinn, NaNa Keum, Edward Giovannucci, Lars T. Fadnes, Paolo Boffetta, Darren C. Greenwood, Serena Tonstad, Lars J. Vatten, Elio Riboli, and Teresa Norat. "Nut consumption and risk of cardiovascular disease, total cancer, all-cause and cause-specific mortality: a systematic review and dose-response meta-analysis of prospective studies." BMC medicine 14, no. 1 (2016): 1-14.

33 Pribis, Peter, and Barbara Shukitt-Hale. "Cognition: the new frontier for nuts and berries." The American journal of clinical nutrition 100, no. suppl_1 (2014): 347S-352S.

34 Aune, Dagfinn, NaNa Keum, Edward Giovannucci, Lars T. Fadnes, Paolo Boffetta, Darren C. Greenwood, Serena Tonstad, Lars J. Vatten, Elio Riboli, and Teresa Norat. "Nut consumption and risk of cardiovascular disease, total cancer, all-cause and cause-specific mortality: a systematic review and dose-response meta-analysis of prospective studies." BMC medicine 14, no. 1 (2016): 1-14.

5 Kim, Yoona, Jennifer Keogh, and Peter M. Clifton. "Nuts and cardio-metabolic disease: A review of meta-analyses." Nutrients 10, no. 12 (2018): 1935.

36 De Souza, Rávila Graziany Machado, Raquel Machado Schincaglia, Gustavo Duarte Pimentel, and João Felipe Mota. "Nuts and human health outcomes: A systematic review." Nutrients 9, no. 12 (2017): 1311.

37 Marventano, Stefano, Maria Izquierdo Pulido, Claudia Sánchez-González, Justyna Godos, Attilio Speciani, Fabio Galvano, and Giuseppe Grosso. "Legume consumption and CVD risk: a systematic review and meta-analysis." Public health nutrition 20, no. 2 (2017): 245-254.

38 Polak, Rani, Edward M. Phillips, and Amy Campbell. "Legumes: Health benefits and culinary approaches to increase intake." Clinical Diabetes 33, no. 4 (2015): 198-205.

39 Aranda-Olmedo, Isabel, and Luis A. Rubio. "Dietary legumes, intestinal microbiota, inflammation and colorectal cancer." Journal of Functional Foods 64 (2020): 103707.

40 Xu, Baojun, and Sam KC Chang. "Comparative study on antiproliferation properties and cellular antioxidant activities of commonly consumed food legumes against nine human cancer cell lines." Food chemistry 134, no. 3 (2012): 1287-1296.

41 Cheah, Irwin K., and Barry Halliwell. "Ergothioneine, recent developments." Redox Biology (2021): 101868.

42 Valverde, María Elena, Talía Hernández-Pérez, and Octavio Paredes-López. "Edible mushrooms: improving human health and promoting quality life." International journal of microbiology 2015 (2015).

43 Mallikarjuna, S. E., A. Ranjini, Devendra J. Haware, M. R. Vijayalakshmi, M. N. Shashirekha, and S. Rajarathnam. "Mineral composition of four edible mushrooms." Journal of Chemistry 2013 (2013).

44 Kalaras, Michael D., John P. Richie, Ana Calcagnotto, and Robert B. Beelman. "Mushrooms: A rich source of the antioxidants ergothioneine and glutathione." Food chemistry 233 (2017): 429-433.

45 Ba, Djibril M., Paddy Ssentongo, Robert B. Beelman, Joshua Muscat, Xiang Gao, and John P. Richie. "Higher Mushroom Consumption Is Associated with Lower Risk of Cancer: A Systematic Review and Meta-Analysis of Observational Studies." Advances in Nutrition (2021).

46 Gargano, Maria Letizia, Leo JLD van Griensven, Omoanghe S. Isikhuemhen, Ulrike Lindequist, Giuseppe Venturella, Solomon P. Wasser, and Georgios I. Zervakis. "Medicinal mushrooms: Valuable biological resources of high exploitation potential." Plant Biosystems-An International Journal Dealing with all Aspects of Plant Biology 151, no. 3 (2017): 548-565.

47 Hall, Kevin D., and Scott Kahan. "Maintenance of lost weight and long-term management of obesity." Medical Clinics 102, no. 1 (2018): 183-197.

Chapter 8

1 Zhang, Zhuoshi, Bernard J. Venn, John Monro, and Suman Mishra. "Subjective satiety following meals incorporating rice, pasta and potato." nutrients 10, no. 11 (2018): 1739.

Index

Acknowledgements

Writing a book is often compared to having a child. As the mom of two human children and now this, my seventh book baby, I can attest they are similar. You pour your mind, body, and soul into a book, albeit more temporary of a focus than for those human types. Because of the time and passion spent, there are several people who supported me immensely during this process, and I want to offer my gratitude.

Thank you to Sharon "Chef Shazzy" Vitullo, who was there through it all: experimenting with recipes, testing and tasting, offering suggestions, and teaching me how to properly say "Worcestershire" with her proper British accent. Eternal gratitude to Catherine Linard for empowering me to choose myself now. Sanford Marcus, thank you for creating with me and for always being fantastically fun, fabulous, and inspiring. To my extraordinary friends Donna Toufer, Kathy Freston, Sheila Small, and Dr. Melanie Joy, who keep me grounded, purposeful, and joyful. Thank you to Ann Barton, my exceptional editor, and Mike Sanders, who supported my vision and made this passion project a reality. Thank you to Marilyn Allen, my fabulous agent, who always has my back and makes things happen. Thank you to my clients who have been open and optimistic, and allowed me into their lives. The concepts outlined in this book unfolded as my education and knowledge from my studies were applied in real life; everything evolved, and I found that science, when mixed with humanity, is quite complex.

About The Author

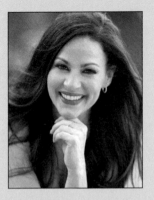

Julieanna Hever, MS, RD, CPT, "The Plant-Based Dietitian" holds a bachelor's degree in theatre and a master's degree in nutrition, bridging her biggest passions for food, presenting, and helping people. She is the host of the *Choose You Now* podcast and has authored six books, including *The Healthspan Solution, Plant-Based Nutrition (Idiot's Guides),* and *The Vegiterranean Diet,* as well as two peer-reviewed journal articles on plant-based nutrition for healthcare professionals. She was the host of *What Would Julieanna Do?,* gave a TEDx talk, and instructed for the eCornell Plant-Based Nutrition Certification Program. She's appeared on *The Dr. Oz Show, Harry,* and *The Steve Harvey Show.* She speaks and consults with clients around the globe. Find her online at ChooseYouNowDiet.com, on Instagram @JulieannaHever, on Facebook @PlantBasedDietitian, and on Twitter @PlantDietitian.